Surgical Treatment of Middle Ear Cholesteatoma

Advances in
Oto-Rhino-Laryngology

Vol. 36

Series Editor
C.R. Pfaltz, Basel

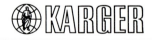

Basel · München · Paris · London · New York · New Delhi · Singapore · Tokyo · Sydney

Surgical Treatment of Middle Ear Cholesteatoma

M. Wayoff, R. Charachon, P. Roulleau, G. Lacher, Ch. Deguine
Translated from the French by *A.N. Baillie*

84 figures and 3 tables, 1987

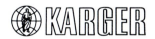

Basel · München · Paris · London · New York · New Delhi · Singapore · Tokyo · Sydney

Advances in Oto-Rhino-Laryngology

Library of Congress Cataloging-in-Publication Data
Traitement chirurgical du cholestéatome de l'oreille moyenne. English. Surgical treatment of
middle ear cholesteatoma
(Advances in oto-rhino-laryngology; vol. 36)
Translation of: Le Traitement chirurgical du cholestéatome de l'oreille moyenne.
Bibliography: p.
Includes index.
1. Cholesteatoma – Surgery. 2. Middle ear – Diseases. I. Wayoff, M. (Michel) II. Title.
III. Series. [DNLM: 1.Cholesteatoma – surgery. 2. Ear, Middle – surgery. W1 AD701 v. 36/WV
200 T766]
RF16.A38 vol. 36 617'.51 s 86-27702
[RF229] [617.8'4059]
ISBN 3-8055-4441-3

Drug Dosage
The authors and the publisher have exerted every effort to ensure that drug selection and dosage set forth in this text are in accord with current recommendations and practice at the time of publication. However, in view of ongoing research, changes in government regulations, and the constant flow of information relating to drug therapy and drug reactions, the reader is urged to check the package insert for each drug for any change in indications and dosage and for added warnings and precautions. This is particularly important when the recommended agent is a new and/or infrequently employed drug.

© Copyright 1987 by S. Karger AG, P.O. Box, CH–4009 Basel (Switzerland)
Printed in Switzerland by gdz (Genossenschaftsdruckerei Zürich)
ISBN 3-8055-4441-3

Contents

Contents

Contents

Preface

Prof. Charachon and his collaborators are to be congratulated for the time and effort involved in preparing this book on cholesteatoma – their English-speaking colleagues are indeed fortunate that they also have had the book translated into English. I was pleased to see that they have considered all of the alternative methods of managing the mastoid. They also clearly differentiate between residual cholesteatoma and recurrent cholesteatoma, and consider in detail various types of iatrogenic cholesteatoma. Their section on results is very interesting, particularly the survey report. Congratulations again on a difficult task well accomplished!

J. Sheehy

Introduction

As early as the beginning of the century, otologists made a distinction, from a clinical point of view, and for the purposes of prognosis and treatment, between antroattic suppuration and tubotympanic suppuration. Cholesteatoma, in its standard form, was of course recognized, but the specific consideration which we today see as necessary had not yet been given to its treatment.

During the first half of the 20th century, the prevention of major complications was otology's real 'raison d'être'. The aim of the 'radical' operations, which were used as a last resort, was to create a considerable marsupialization of the tympanic and mastoid cavities into the external auditory canal. In order to avoid the deleterious effect of such operations on the hearing, they were only indicated when certain warning signs were present. A few authors spoke of the necessity to sacrifice hearing. Nowadays, it must be recognized that the need to give the patient objective information does pose problems. It is still necessary now, as then, to use such terse and cogent arguments as 'it's better to be alive and deaf than to die with perfect hearing'.

A few surgeons, however, who were already concerned to avoid needless mutilation, suggested the use of 'modified' or 'partial' radical operations. One of these surgeons was Sourdille [226] who wrote, in his thesis, of the radical mastoidectomy: 'The poor results, from a functional point of view, made a reaction inevitable.' Surgery at that time had only one aim to halt the process and favour healing. Sourdille [226] then asked the four essential questions which are still important today about the surgical treatment: (1) What is the necessary anatomical modification? (2) How, in view of the lesions, can it heal then? (3) When then lesions have healed, can there be a further improvement? (4) Is cholesteatoma to be considered as a complication which necessarily involves radical surgery? These four questions have been answered in various ways over the years, as our knowledge of the physiopathology of the lesions on the one hand, and the instruments at our disposal on the other, have both improved.

Heath, Bondy and then Sourdille [226] already thought that cholesteatoma helped rather than hindered epithelialization. From then on, compromise solutions were necessary, although major complications were still common enough to be the predominant factor in the indication for surgery. The main aim was to exenterate the antromastoid cavities, leaving intact all those elements in the tympanic cavity which were functional, and either preserving the fibrous annulus (Heath, 1906 – modified radical operation), or sacrificing it (Bondy, 1908). The state of the tympanic cavity was thus already the determining factor in deciding whether a conservative approach was to be used or not.

These remained the basic principles of otology until the introduction of antibiotics and, as is always the case when ideas and attitudes are changing, this period of transition was also a period of stagnation, as stragglers caught up with the new techniques and primature enthusiam inevitably waned. The swing of the pendulum is, moreover, apparent in the changing attitudes of each individual surgeon, and it is thus rare to find unanimity at any one time. Let us take, for example, the term 'atticitis' which is still, unfortunately, for some surgeons a concept which is independent of cholesteatoma. This is not, however, a harmless mistake since, in the words of Aristotle, 'the concept "dog" does not bite'. We have all seen cholesteatomas, labelled 'atticitis', develop without any real treatment.

The introduction of antibiotics opened a new era especially from the clinical point of view, while progress in surgery is more due to the use of the surgical microscope and improved instruments. By controlling most of the infectious phenomena, antibiotics have made it possible for us to appreciate the fundamental importance of the presence or absence of keratinizing, desquamating stratum malpighii in the middle ear cavities. By halting the development of acute otitis media in most cases, they have made it possible to demonstrate that inflammation of the tympanic and mastoid cavities almost invariably precedes the infection. It is thus possible to demonstrate the complexity of the pathogenesis of chronic otitis media, which is dependent on so many factors that it is difficult to analyze them all at the same time in such a way as to obtain an overall view.

In the 1966 report to the French ENT Association, it was shown that there are many different possible relationships between the different anatomico-clinical varieties of chronic otitis media. The formation of the lesions depends on biochemical, bacteriological and mechanical factors. Their appearance depends on the involvement in the inflammatory process of the mucosa, the connective tissue, the bone and the epithelium respectively. As techniques developed, so did the classification of chronic otitis media, although there was no specific therapeutic approach to cholesteatoma.

Developments in Technique

Developments in technique took place continually as experience was gained. It was not long, however, before the major types of indication became clear: sequelae or conditions assessed as such, simple chronic otitis media, and chronic otitis media with cholesteatoma. The introduction of tympanoplasty by Wullstein and Zollner was certainly the result of antibiotics, the microscope and audiometry. The maintenance or restoration of hearing was seen as a challenge. As from 1960, after a short, abortive, period when skin grafts were used, new developments were again made in technique – connective tissue was favoured for repairing the tympanic membrane, the ossicles were transposed or replaced, and then tympano-ossicular homografts were used. Such progress is not of course made without moments of transition and hesitation. A certain degree of hindsight is necessary, for example, to see that progressive sensorineural impairment is too often observed after stapedectomy for tympanosclerosis, or that residual cholesteatomas are frequent after reconstructive surgery without second look. The value of the operation is not denied, but we must avoid its becoming discredited through incorrect indications.

Developments in Attitude

With experience, it was possible to understand certain important points. From the functional point of view, the ideal aim is to leave the tympano-ossicular system intact, or to reconstruct it, keeping the anatomical structure as close as possible to normal – whence the importance of keeping the whole bony canal intact, and having a flexible tympanic membrane. No reconstruction of the tympano-ossicular system can remain stable in the long term unless the middle ear cavities (tympanic and mastoid cavities) are adequately ventilated. Surgeons thus became increasingly conscious of the importance of the physiology of the Eustachian tube which is still, in fact, not totally understood. During this period, surgical theory gave pride of place to the contents of the ear. Sourdille wrote (and this was not contested until recent years): 'When we look properly at the middle ear we see that it has only two constituent parts – the container, i.e. the bony shell ... and the contents, the tympanic membrane and the ossicular chain, the noble part, which alone is functional.' The progress which has been made from the conceptual point of view is to have understood that the 'container' is equally important, and that the contents cannot function in any lasting way unless they are protected and aerated. There are two aspects to the middle ear – hearing and aeration. Hearing will be affected, sooner or later, by any dysfunction in aeration. The challenge today is thus to restore the ear in its entirety. Ventilation of the middle ear cavities by physiological means can only be through the Eustachian tube. This is the ideal which must be aimed at, aeration of a cavity through the meatus being only a poor second best.

Furthermore, with the benefit of hindsight, the inadequacies of the different techniques were seen:

(A) Atticoantrostomy, in our view, has no place in this context. Historically, it was introduced after the partial mastoidectomy. The name is in fact ambiguous and has been misunderstood by many otologists, leading, in the not so distant past, to operations which were often incomplete and iatrogenic. Cholesteatoma requires a specific therapeutic strategy, in which there is no place for surgery 'as required by the lesions', which is often carried out from in front backwards, preserving the bony annulus. Such operations only led to false drainage and inadequate aeration, generally without being able to prevent the recurrence of cholesteatoma growth in those areas left intact.

(B) Partial mastoidectomy does not prevent recurrence in the tympanic cavity.

(C) Obliteration is an attempt to settle this problem. Moscher had the idea as early as 1911. In 1962, Palva [154] gave this name to this method of managing the posterior cavity. In France, Bouche et al. [23] drew up the list of the main indications for obliteration techniques. In fact, many authors are reluctant to use obliteration, fearing the risk of a residual cholesteatoma developing undetected under the obliteration.

(D) Conchoplasty, in the view of some authors, is a means of adapting the size of the meatus to the volume of the operation cavity. In 1966, in the Report to the French ENT Association, entitled 'Stages in the Treatment of Chronic Otitis Media in Adults', the problem posed by the bony surface of a marsupialized mastoid cavity was stressed. When the cavity is large, epithelialization is rarely stable in the long term. The result is better if the bone has reacted to the cholesteatoma matrix, i.e. when the mastoid is eburned or when closed-technique surgery is later transformed into an open technique. Especially in children, however, a cholesteatoma may very well be present with a highly pneumatized mastoid. The self-cleansing cavity may be attained by 'saucerization'. For the mastoid, an 'all-or-nothing' rule has been suggested by one of the present authors [254]. There can be no half measures when exenterating the mastoid – the slightest cleft, or a single air cell which has been left, will sooner or later make its presence known. If the mastoid is very highly pneumatized, exenteration may seem impossible, and surgery must very often be revised. Although most reports give a figure of 70% of stable cavities, regular, life-long follow-up and inspection is always necessar, and the cavity must be cleaned at least annually.

Maintaining the anatomical independence of the aerated tympanic and mastoid cavities by preserving the posterior canal wall and repairing the tympanic membrane is the other half of this alternative, the 'to be or not to be' of the mastoid. In 1958, Jansen [113] suggested that posterior tympanotomy could provide a combined transmastoid and transcanal approach to the cholesteatoma. In France, in 1968, Sterkers [230] set the style when he spoke of 'reconstructive cholesteatectomy'. In Belgium, Marquet [138] had already suggested that tympano-ossicular homografts would make it possible to remove the lesions more thoroughly. Wullstein [259], of course, and then Antoli-Candella [12], had already had the idea of exploring the posterior part of the tympanic cavity by opening an orifice between the facial nerve and the bony annulus, but Jansen must take the credit for suggesting an ordered, extensive approach to the posterior tympanum. Proctor [173] had already described all the clefts in which epidermis could remain concealed in this area. In the English-speaking countries, this extremely conservative attitude was adopted by Sheehy [202], and by

Smyth [223]. In France, Portmann [169] suggested the term 'closed technique', equivalent to the English abbreviations CAT and ICWT (see below).

After some years, there were protests at the frequency with which cholesteatomas were recurring from retraction pockets on the one hand, and from residual epithelium on the other hand, as a result of incomplete removal. Some surgeons therefore, like Smyth [222], went back completely to the open technique; others, like Austin [13], distinguished between the indications for the two techniques, and frequently changed to an open technique at a second stage of the operation. Sheehy [215], Marquet [245] and especially Jansen [110] still favour, except in special cases, the preservation and restoration involved in the closed techniques. For most surgeons who support this method, a routine second look – i.e. a second stage of the operation – is essential, making it possible either to change to an open technique, or to keep to a closed technique after treating the residual lesion or the recurrence, while it may be mecessary in certain exceptional cases, to envisage a third stage to check on results.

Over the last 5 or 6 years, otological conferences have been the scene of discussions, some of them quite passionate, in which a contrast is drawn between the cost of repeated surgery and the desire to improve hearing and between the technical difficulties and the need to spread the use of the technique. At the instigation of J.Sade, two International Conferences on Cholesteatoma and Mastoid Surgery have been held, at Iowa City in 1976 and Tel Aviv in 1981. Our aim is to take stock of this very controversial question, referring to our own experience and the more important statistics of those of our colleagues who were kind enough to reply to our questionnaire.

If closed techniques are so much in vogue at present, this is because the aim they seek to achieve is compatible with thorough, modern surgical techniques. Does the improvement in hearing come up to this aim? Is it justifiable to take a calculated risk and leave a residual cholesteatoma in place? Does preservation of the canal really make it possible to practice a sport in normal conditions, and if necessary to wear a hearing aid? Are open techniques really one hundred percent safe? Is it more economic to look after cavities which have become destabilized than to perform second-look surgery? What are the overall results from a functional point of view? Should individual considerations (i.e. the treatment of the individual as an individual) be systematically sacrificed in favour of statistical theories which, it must be stressed, vary enormously?

Let us say, in the words of D. Plester, that if we use all sorts of techniques against the cholesteatoma, even those which are the 'last word' in surgery, all too often the cholesteatoma itself will have 'the last word'. We therefore refuse to take up any categorical attitude, in the conviction that any conclusion reached can only be a provisional one until our basic physiopathological knowledge is improved.

Definitions

Definition of Cholesteatoma

From a therapeutic point of view, we shall consider that there is a cholesteatoma whenever collections of more or less organized epithelial cells are permanently present inside the normal plane of the tympanic membrane, which may be perforated or more or less invaginated – in other words, as Gray says, when there is 'skin in the wrong place'. In the first chapter, we shall look at all the macroscopic and microscopic aspects of the cholesteatoma, and the reactions in the structures which it invades.

For many years cholesteatoma was only diagnosed, and surgery was only envisaged, when the otoscopic picture was evident. Today, the treatment of cholesteatoma must include an element of prevention which implies a good understanding of the pathogenesis of the cholesteatoma and of the physiopathology of the middle ear. We have therefore devoted quite a long chapter to this subject in the hope that it may spur the reader on to think more deeply about the matter.

For the clinical point of view, diagnosis is generally simple. Unfortunately, the use of the microscope during consultation has not yet become routine, and too many errors are still made in assessing the lesions. Precursors of cholesteatoma are given too little attention, and intermediate stages are not always noticed. The value of microscopic cleaning of the canal is underrated, and it is too seldom used. We shall give precise definitions for the terms 'epidermosis', 'retraction or invagination pockets', 'epithelialization of the tympanic cavity', 'sac cholesteatoma' and 'finger-shaped cholesteatoma'. Although some otoscopic features are pathognomonic, it must be stressed that, whatever the appearance of the tympanic membrane, the possibility of an epithelial invasion can never be dismissed. For example, a tongue of epithelium, which may become active and start progressing at any moment, may be attached to the medial surface of a tympanosclerosis plaque of apparently innocent appearance, at the edge of a perforation which has long been dry. Although the specialized otologist may be familiar with all the different facets of cholesteatoma, he must also be able to detect dangerous forms which may lead to complications – a subject to which we devote a special chapter.

From the point of view of treatment, the treatment of functional sequelae gives rise to a certain number of iatrogenic cholesteatomas, when a fragment of epithelium in the tympanic cavity is not seen, or when such a fragment is buried during surgery. We shall also consider the difference between recurrent and residual cholesteatomas. Although the latter are particularly linked to closed techniques, the former can occur after any type of surgery.

Surgical Techniques

Fleury et al. [77] have on several occasions stressed the importance of the precise use of terminology when speaking of the surgery of chronic otitis media. The number of different terms which have been used since the end of the last century is impressive, and the vocabulary of the subject has become diversified in differing degrees, depending on the country and the language involved. It must nonetheless be acknowledged that, since the introduction of antibiotics, ideas on strategy have become clearer. As Fleury et al. put it: 'in former times, it was enough for some surgeons to make a small opening from the masto-antro-attic cavities into the canal to allow drainage... Such cavities were often made by surgeons who were afraid to close the cavities completely, for fear of shutting in the disease, but who did not dare to perform a radical mastoidectomy either'. Experience has shown that these half open techniques are often iatrogenic – in the ear, the surgeon's sins are not always immediately punished, so that inadequate operations may appear to be partly successful. A cholesteatoma may thus develop in an ear which should have remained healthy. In simple cases of chronic otitis media, we have thus seen the gradual disappearance of the more or less typical transcanal atticotomies, with or without preservation of the bony annulus. When a cholesteatoma is present, there is an absolute need to choose between preserving or sacrificing the whole of the bony envelope. Mucosa and skin can only be juxtaposed. In the words of Bremond and Magnan [25]. 'In this disease where skin and mucosa are opponents', a surgeon who performs a radical mastoidectomy 'deliberately takes the side of the skin and sacrifices the mucosa – this means the elimination of the middle ear, which must be followed by the epithelialization of that cavity. It is a good plan, but difficult to carry out'.

Like Portmann [169] therefore, we shall make a distinction between two main groups: open technique and closed technique.

Open Technique or Canal-Down Technique

Complete Radical Mastoidectomy. This is the standard, classical radical mastoidectomy, unmitigatedly radical, both in the complete evacuation of the contents and in the regular shaping of the walls. It gives a spherical cavity with 'saucerized', edges, to use M. Paparella's term. It naturally involves the attic and antrum if the mastoid is compact and the antrum is the only existing cell. Only one attitude can be adopted towards the facial ridge – it must be completely lowered in its posterior, lateral and anterior portions.

Open Technique with Management of the Tympanic Cavity. As Sourdille [226] wrote, the state of the tympanic cavity must be the deciding factor as to whether or not to adopt a conservative procedure. Today we should rather say a reparative procedure. There is indeed no question of leaving the tympanic cavity open above, if we do not wish to see the cholesteatoma recurring at some later date behind the preserved pars tensa, as was the case in many atticotomies or partial mastoidectomies. The 'management' of the cavity means the construction of a 'tympanum' with or without a columellar effect. This is a 'modified radical mastoidectomy' and can only be envisaged nowadays with an associated tympanoplasty.

Open Technique with 'Management' of the Tympanic and Posterior cavities. A musculoperiosteal flap (Palva) is added to the preceding operation, in order both to reduce the size of the cavity and to stabilize epithelialization. This is what Smyth calls the MOT mastoid obliteration with tympanoplasty after previous mastoidectomy.

Meatoconchoplasty is another type of management of the posterior cavity, adapting the aeration to the volume of the cavity.

Closed Technique or Canal-Up Technique

The most important characteristic of this type of operation is the fact that the posterior canal wall and the outer attic wall are either left intact or reconstructed as perfectly as possible. In the latter case, the reconstruction may be carried out during the first stage of the operation by removing and immediately replacing the outer attic wall [259] or the posterior canal wall [67, 68].

For most authors, the closed technique involves no terminological ambiguity. There is no doubt that the use of the term implies an attempt to perform a 'cholesteatectomy' by a combined transcanal and transmastoid approach. The ideal solution is to approach the cholesteatoma from behind by opening the mastoid wide, to dissect it and to push it completely towards the tympanic cavity through the posterior tympanotomy. As Fisch [72] has stressed, the mastoidectomy, which is essential, must remove the cells as thoroughly as possible, with the same rules as for a radical mastoidectomy, except that the posterior bony wall of the external auditory meatus need necessarily be left intact. After removal of the cholesteatoma, the tympanic membrane, and perhaps the ossicular chain, are repaired in various ways (standard rules for tympanoplasty).

Closed technique may be called combined approach tympanoplasty (CAT) [217] or intact canal wall tympanoplasty (ICWT) [203]. In fact, neither term includes the essential step in these operations: Jansen's posterior tympanotomy. In a special chapter, we shall deal in great detail with the technique and difficulty of this all-important manoeuvre on which the effectiveness of the operation depends. In our view, the fact that this step is not mentioned in the nomenclature may have one essential consequence – the step ist too often avoided by inexperienced surgeons or those who are unsure of themselves. The fact that the quality of a closed technique depends above all on the posterior tympanotomy can never be overemphasized. All the preliminary steps in the operation (approach route, opening of the mastoid, freeing of the canal skin, perhaps drilling of the canal) are planned with a view to the three (epi-, meso- and hypotympanic) steps of the posterior tympanotomy.

Pathology

Macroscopic Appearances

Cholesteatoma is defined as the presence of skin in the middle ear, with an accumulation of keratin forming a benign tumour, which some surgeons prefer to call a keratoma. But it is also necessary to include a less well-defined aspect – the presence of skin in the middle ear, without the retention of keratin – which we shall refer to as epithelialization of the tympanic cavity. There are also rarer forms such as closed tympanic membrane cholesteatomas, cholesteatomas of the canal and intrapetrous extensions of cholesteatomas of the middle ear. After the macroscopic aspects, we shall look at the microscopic aspects and reactions to the cholesteatoma in the surrounding bone, ossicles, labyrinth and facial nerve, and their histogenesis. A special section will be devoted to iatrogenic cholesteatomas.

Typical Cholesteatoma

The simplest definition is 'skin in the wrong place'. The skin desquamates and the product of this desquamation forms a pseudo-tumour which develops off-centre and usually becomes infected. This skin, without appendages, is called the matrix and has a characteristically shiny appearance. It is the essential element which produces the cholesteatoma and determines how far it will extend. This greasy appearance of the desquamated mass (J. Muller) gave rise to the name 'cholesteatoma' which is in fact a misnomer, and a source of confusion histopathologically, with the cholesterol granuloma, which is a very different thing.

Current techniques in tympanoplasty require the total removal of the cholesteatoma. This requirement has considerably increased our knowledge of its propagation. The cholesteatoma may start from one

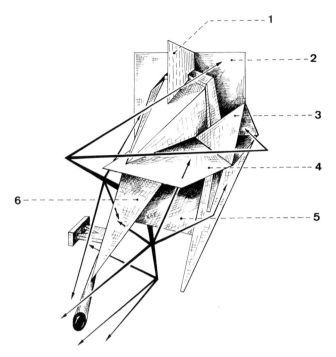

Fig. 1. Schematic posterior view of the mucosal folds and ligaments of the middle ear (after Proctor). 1 = Superior ligament of the malleus; 2 = Superior malleolar ligament; 3 = lateral ligament of the malleus; 4 = lateral ligament of the incus; 5 = interossicular ligament; 6 = incudostapedial ligament. Arrows show the cholesteatoma progression.

of two zones – the region of the pars flaccida or the region of the pars tensa. In the latter case the cholesteatoma is associated with those lesions which will be described with the epithelialization of the tympanum. Let us stress that in the vast majority of cholesteatomas there is an anatomical continuity between the matrix and the skin of the external auditory meatus and of the tympanic membrane. From its starting point, cholesteatoma moulds itself to the pre-existing elements, and goes round obstacles before it destroys them. It travels by the preformed pathways between the ossicles and the mucosal folds and ligaments of the attic, which Proctor [173–175] has so well described. Marquet [139–140] has shown the progress diagrammatically (fig. 1).

It is tempting to say that the cholesteatoma develops differently depending on the surrounding bone [36]. In a sclerotic bone, it forms a regular, rounded mass, with sometimes one or two lobe-like extensions towards the tympanic cavity or the Eustachian tube. In a pneumatized bone, on the other hand, there will be many epithelial ingrowths, joined by thin pedicles to the main mass. In fact, however, a cholesteatoma may erode a hard eburnated bone, pushing layered extensions into the slightest gap. Again, in a pneumatized bone, a regular-shaped cholesteatoma sac may remain at a distance from one or several walls. It is very difficult to determine the reasons for this difference in the bone structure. Was there no pneumatization prior to the development of the cholesteatoma? Or is the reason not rather the speed at which the cholesteatoma develops? If growth is slow, the bone has time to react and become more dense; if it is rapid, the cholesteatoma is pushed into the air cells, and if the bone then reacts, epidermic fragments may be surrounded and appear to be isolated. We may thus describe two macroscopic appearances – the hernial sac cholesteatoma and the extensive cholesteatoma.

Hernial Sac Cholesteatoma

This seems to develop slowly. It may extend considerably, particularly in certain zones.

Attic

All cholesteatomas must pass through the attic. If they start from the pars flaccida, they may remain confined to the lateral attic, clinging closely to the ossicular chain. They erode the lateral attic wall, which may be completely destroyed (fig. 2). If the cholesteatoma grows upwards from the mesotympanum, it may occupy only the medial attic, internal to the incus, the horizontal process of which it may surround, or internal to the head of the malleus, passing either behind or in front of the tensor tympani tendon. It may then pass forwards into the root of the zygoma from the supra-tubal recess or towards the geniculate ganglion. The ossicles are affected to a greater or lesser extent (fig. 3).

Antrum

The cholesteatoma sac swells in the aditus and develops gradually in the antrum. The cholesteatoma sometimes only occupies the ante-

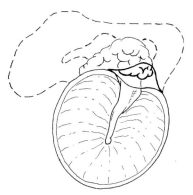

Fig. 2. Sac cholesteatoma in the lateral attic. This generally forms from an invagination of the pars flaccida. The notch of Rivinus is always osteitic. The outer attic wall may be amputated.

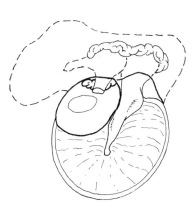

Fig. 3. Sac cholesteatoma in the medial attic. This generally forms from a posterior subligamentary invagination, then passes medially to the incus and the head of the malleus. Often, as here, it destroys the long process of the incus and the superstructure of the stapes.

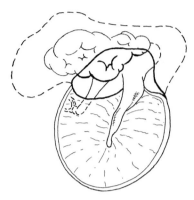

Fig. 4. Sac cholesteatoma in attic and antrum. The sac does not necessarily adhere to the posterior wall of the antrum. The body of the incus and the head of the malleus may be partially or totally destroyed while the handle of the malleus and the long process of the incus provide normal hearing if they are still joined by the inferior part of the incudomallear joint.

rior half of the antrum without reaching the posterior wall, adhering to a greater or lesser degree to the superior, medial and lateral walls (fig. 4). Even at this stage in its development, it may have opened a fistula in the lateral or even the superior semicircular canal, especially if it has developed in an eburnated bone. In such cases it is not possible to eliminate the mechanism of compression-erosion. From the antrum, the cholesteatoma may migrate downwards and forwards, itself opening a posterior tympanotomy, threatening the lateral semicircular canal and the facial nerve. There is a high risk of fistula in these cases.

Mastoid

The cholesteatoma bulges to a greater or lesser extent into the mastoid and may go as far as the tip (fig. 5). It is practically always possible to determine a plane of cleavage, except sometimes at the meninges or the lateral sinus where the cholesteatoma matrix is tightly adherent. Sometimes a low dura may make it difficult to approach the posterosuperior angle of this mastoid cavity (Citelli's sinodural angle). Usually the difficulty is not here because after the cholesteatoma has been dissected, the mastoid may be drilled again, removing a consider-

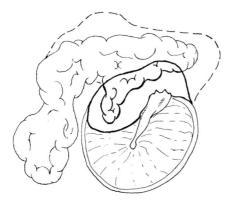

Fig. 5. Sac cholesteatoma in attic, antrum and mastoid, with posterior extension into the tympanic cavity. The cholesteatoma may reach as far as the tip of the mastoid. It forms a mass in the posterior part of the tympanic cavity, migrating towards the round window. This mass sometimes erodes the facial recess, threatening the lateral semicircular canal and the facial nerve.

able thickness of bone, going well beyond the cholesteatoma matrix, thus ensuring that the removal has been thorough.

Mesotympanum

If it descends from the attic, the cholesteatoma forms a mass which is generally posterior, between the facial ridge which it erodes to a greater or lesser extent and the cochleariform process, destroying the long process of the incus and the superstructure of the stapes. It often does not reach as far as the footplate from which it is separated by granulomatous tissue or a layer of connective tissue. If the superstructure of the stapes is intact, the cholesteatoma will still adhere to it but the sac can be fairly easily detached (fig. 6). This mass often descends towards the round window, moulding itself to the retrotympanum hidden by the overhang of the posterior sulcus. This retrotympanum forms a groove [9, 11, 58, 91, 100, 101, 174] which is difficult to get behind the round window. Only an inferiorly extended posterior tympanotomy, or complete lowering of the facial ridge can provide adequate access. In this area, the cholesteatoma sometimes extends on either side of the facial nerve. Laterally, it involves the facial recess – medially, it may enter the sinus tympani, between the pyramidal pro-

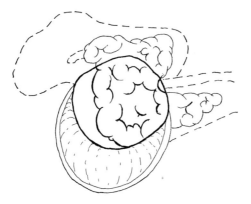

Fig. 6. Sac cholesteatoma in attic and antrum, passing forwards in the tympanic cavity, with a lobe pushing into the Eustachian tube. If the lobe is not broken, this extension into the Eustachian tube can be fairly easily dissected.

cess and the facial nerve laterally and the ampulla of the posterior semicircular canal medially (fig. 7). In such cases it is generally possible to find a plane of cleavage and remove this invagination in toto, but it is often necessary to remove the pyramidal process and the superior part of the stapes muscle after skeletonizing the facial nerve. Sometimes the cholesteatoma extends to the beginning of the infralabyrinthine cell tract, in the posterior recess of the hypotympanum, which is definitely the weak point in the posterior part of the tympanic cavity. Such an extension may necessitate the opening of an approach between the facial nerve and the sigmoid sinus, inferior to the labyrinth.

In the hypotympanum itself, dissection is very difficult, as the cholesteatoma passes between the cells in this area and adheres to the cell walls. Dissection must alternate with drilling, using a diamond burr and taking care not to tear the jugular bulb.

When the cholesteatoma has developed from an epithelialization of the mesotympanum, the lesions are particulary complex. The skin adheres closely to the bone, clings to or destroys the superstructure of the stapes, enters the facial recess, the sinus tympani and the cells of the hypotympanum. The plane of cleavage, which is usually found

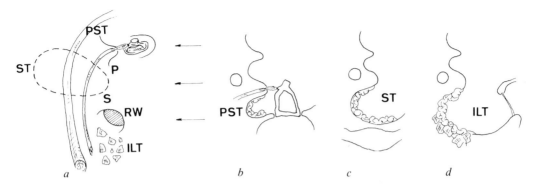

Fig. 7. Cholesteatoma invading the internal retrotympanum. *a* Area of the internal retrotympanum (RW = round window; P = ponticulus; S = subiculum; PST = posterior sinus tympani; ST = sinus tympani; ILT = infralabyrinthine tract). *b* Superior section: posterior sinus tympani (PST). *c* Middle section: sinus tympani (ST). *d* Inferior section: infralabyrinthine tract (ILT)

around lobes of the cholesteatoma migrating from below upwards, is generally nonexistent, and there is a much greater risk that the dissection will be inadequate.

Tympanic Membrane

Wherever it may have originated, the cholesteatoma often progresses downwards and forwards, either under the edge of a posterior perforation or behind an apparently healthy tympanic membrane. Generally the cholesteatoma sac can be dissected from the tympanic membrane. Sometimes, however, it will infiltrate the medial surface, disrupting the fibres of the pars tensa. Dissection is impossible and the whole suspect zone must be removed. Sometimes, on the other hand, the cholesteatoma produces large lobes within the mesotympanum without adhering to its walls.

Eustachian Tube

The orifice of the Eustachian tube may be affected when there are massive invasions from the tympanic cavity or from a cholesteatoma in the anterior attic. This is generally a perfectly limited, encapsulated extension, which can be dissected without breaking the matrix. The Eustachian tube is then revealed to be perfectly healthy. Sometimes, however, the pocket is broken inside the tube and, although the anterior sulcus has been eliminated, it is very difficult to check how far the cholesteatoma extends into the Eustachian tube. Another possibility, especially in cases of epithelialization of the mesotympanum, is that the Eustachian tube may become blocked by tympanosclerosis or hyperostosis. Such pathology must be drilled away very carefully, using a diamond burr, because of the proximity of the internal carotid artery. In short, the sac cholesteatoma, which is limited and self-contained, can in general be dissected very accurately. If, however, the cholesteatoma has been developing over a long period, there may be extensions into areas which are more difficult to get at and to check. It must be stressed that such difficulties are most often found in the tympanic cavity, especially when the cholesteatoma has developed from an epithelialization of the mesotympanum.

Finger-Like Cholesteatoma

Also known as a ramified cholesteatoma. The unorganized nature of its development often seems to be determined by the degree of infection and of maceration. Here again, the pneumatization of the mastoid often plays a part, especially in children. In other cases, the cholesteatoma produces layered, medial extensions, which form, medially to the labyrinth, more massive growths within an extreme densification of the petrous bone which may suggest the presence of a primary cholesteatoma. The histopathological appearance, perhaps more often than with sac cholesteatomas, is papillary, because of the wrinkling of the basal layer, which detaches epidermic cones from along the vessels in its underlying bone and forms epithelial digitations in the chorion.

Finger-Like Cholesteatoma in a Pneumatized Mastoid (fig. 8)

The lobes of the cholesteatoma pass from cell to cell at a distance from the main mass. They may reach the meninges and the wall of the lateral sinus. Wullstein [257] mentions a problem which we have also encountered – the cholesteatoma may enter a fissure and appear to terminate there, whereas in fact it is developing, concealed, between the medial surface of the temporal bone and the meninges or the lateral sinus. This is the type of cholesteatoma which may fill the tympanic cavity and extend into the Eustachian tube. They often reach the

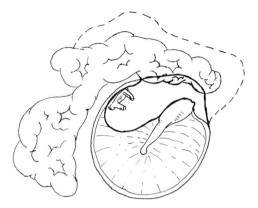

Fig. 8. Finger-like cholesteatoma in pneumatized mastoid. The lobes of the cholesteatoma develop irregularly from cell to cell. A routine search must be made for extensions which go even further.

hypotympanum, where their lobes may penetrate the cells of the hypotympanic recess. This may be more of these cells than expected, and
eradication will be particularly difficult. When dissecting the cholesteatoma from the medial wall of the middle ear, the surgeon must
check every invagination into the cells, and look specially at the four
cell tracts where the fingers of these cholesteatomas are usually found.

The anterior supralabyrinthine tract passes above the second portion of the facial nerve, in front of the ampulla of the superior semicircular canal. An extension of the cholesteatoma may enter the cells in
this tract. This type of propagation may easily be verified by meticulous dissection, alternating with drilling with a diamond burr, being
very careful not to damage the facial nerve and the superior semicircular canal. The cholesteatoma may indeed have exposed the facial nerve
and opened the ampulla of the superior semicircular canal. In some
cases, the cholesteatoma here disappears, passing medially to the ampulla of the semicircular canal and developing medially to the vestibule, forming an intrapetrous cholesteatoma which requires a middle
fossa approach.

The translabyrinthine cell tract begins above the lateral semicircular canal and follows the vestige of the petromastoid canal inside the
concavity of the superior semicircular canal. The cholesteatoma may

send out an extension which can be controlled, or go beyond the curve of the canal to develop in contact with the internal auditory canal, requiring a middle fossa approach unless hearing has already been destroyed.

The posterior supralabyrinthine cell tract passes posterior to the superior semicircular canal, and superior to the posterior semicircular canal. It is common to find a cholesteatoma hernia in this tract. It only becomes impossible to control through the otological approach when the cholesteatoma extends medially to the posterior or superior semicircular canal. Here again, a middle fossa approach must be used, unless the hearing has been destroyed in which case a posterior translabyrinthine approach is possible.

The disposition of the infralabyrinthine cell tract varies greatly depending on the height of the jugular bulb. The most anterior cells follow the internal carotid below the cochlea. Dissection with a blunt needle and drilling with a diamond burr suffice to deal with this type of extension if it is limited. The most posterior cells are medial to the facial nerve in the area of the posterior recess of the hypotympanum, a frontier zone situated inferior to the sinus tympani. This is a definite weak point [39] in the tympanic cavity, under the posterior labyrinth (fig. 9). Here, the cholesteatoma may send out an extension medial to the facial nerve, inferior to the ampulla of the posterior semicircular canal and superior to the bulb of the internal jugular. It can generally be removed by opening a infralabyrinthine approach between the facial nerve and the sigmoid sinus. When the extension is larger it may open a path for itself between the internal carotid in front and the jugular bulb behind, going on towards the tip of the petrous bone, possibly destroying the cochlea or part of the posterior labyrinth. In such cases it is necessary to use an infratemporal approach, re-routing the second and third portions of the facial nerve.

Finger-Like Cholesteatoma in Eburnated Mastoid

The cholesteatoma enters the remaining spongy bone around the labyrinth. Here again, it extends along the four main directions taken by the intrapetrous cell tracts which we have just seen. But the speed of penetration is different; it proceeds layer by layer, surrounded by obvious bone reconstruction, sometimes forming irregular blocks, covered by a thin layer of epidermis. Sometimes the bone reconstruction has a massive appearance, which Fleury [76] calls the osteomatous

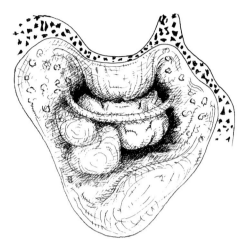

Fig. 9. Extension of cholesteatoma to facial recess and posterior weak point of the tympanic cavity. This weak point consists of the posterior recess of the hypotympanum at the beginning of the posterior infralabyrinthine cell tract.

form. In some cases, the contrast between this far-reaching extension and the scarcity of the cholesteatoma in the attic suggest that this sort of cholesteatoma is primary.

Cholesteatoma in Children

Cholesteatomas seem to extend very rapidly in children. There are two possible explanations for this – the speed of tissue growth and the degree of infection and inflammation brought by the Eustachian tube. Growth of tissue is much faster in children than in adults. Inflammation (seromucous otitis) or infection (suppuration) is much commoner than in adults. The cholesteatoma develops rapidly in a pneumatized mastoid which it 'takes by surprise' and which has no time to react other than by suppuration or the formation of a cholesterol granuloma. All these factors explain the extensive, finger-like shape taken by cholesteatomas in children and the fact that it usually extends to the mesotympanum, which is the point of least resistance, and particularly subject to inflammation originating in the Eustachian tube with seromucous effusion [37, 110, 116, 201, 207]. In some cases, however, the mastoid is eburnated, and the cholesteatoma fills small bone cavities which it erodes, retaining at the same time its ability to extend to the mesotympanum and even the Eustachian tube.

Epidermization of the Middle Ear

The definition which Schuknecht [197] gives of epidermization is clear – replacement of the mucosa by squamous keratinizing epithelium, without retention of keratin debris. In our view, two aspects can be separated – the first, known in recent years as epidermosis, is a more or less disorderly migration of epidermis. The second, which has become better known through observation of seromucous otitis, is the fixed retraction pocket.

Epidermosis
The term 'epidermosis' should be confined to migrations of epidermis, in a sheet or a mass, from a protruding or adhering part, and particularly the handle of the malleus. The handle of the malleus at the centre of a perforation may thus be extended by a 'horn' or tube of skin, which sometimes reaches the hypotympanum at its other extremity. It may also adhere to the promontory, serving to guide the gradual progress of a strip of epidermis with a scalloped edge, which may be fairly stable, or which may develop quickly on the promontory if there is inflammation (fig. 10). An embossed appearance is often caused by thickening over a protruding pearl of tympanosclerosis at the edge of the perforation. Less noticeably, the epidermis may pass from the edge of the perforation on to the chorda tympani and from there to the inferior process of the incus, going on to cover the stapes, its tendon and sometimes the surrounding areas (fig. 11). It may be said that epidermosis is the current stage in the theory of direct migration. In some cases, however, these phenomena are quite considerable and may lead to a cholesteatoma, and to difficulties, comparable to those caused by fixed retraction pockets. In other cases the epithelium is separated from the promontory by a clear plane of dissection, supported by a very thin veil of fibrous tissue, which forms a sort of spider's web invaginated into the tympanic cavity, on to which the epithelium has passed. Dissection is safe and rapid.

The epidermis sometimes passes on to the medial surface of the tympanic membrane, either from a traumatic perforation, or via a

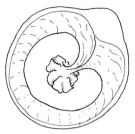

Fig. 10. Typical epidermosis developing on the promontory from contact with the inferior end of the handle of the malleus.

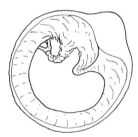

Fig. 11. Epidermosis passing from the edge of a perforation onto the inferior process of the incus and going on to cover the stapes, its tendon, and sometimes the surrounding areas.

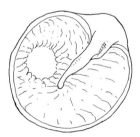

Fig. 12. Epidermosis migrating to the medial surface of the tympanic membrane. The epidermis is guided by the thickening of the edge of the perforation which is infiltrated by tympanosclerosis. This epidermic migration may also be caused by a tear in the tympanic membrane, of traumatic origin, with eversion of a flap on its surface.

thickened ledge of tympanosclerosis, guiding the epidermis towards the medial surface of the tympanic membrane which it follows for several millimetres (fig. 12). By dissecting the tympanosclerosis plaque supporting the epidermis, or by everting the tympanic membrane, it is generally possible to see the scalloped edge of this epidermis. Sometimes the edge is lost from view around the annulus and, even though all the remaining parts of the tympanic membrane and the surrounding mucosa have been removed, it is never possible to be sure that the removal of the epidermis has been complete.

Fixed Retraction Pockets

We are not concerned here with retraction pockets which can be elevated by insufflation or the insertion of an air tube in the tympanic membrane. We are rather concerned with retraction pockets in which the epidermis replaces the mucosa of the middle ear. The stratum Malpighii lies directly on the chorion which is often extremely thin. Dissection must be at the level of the bony surface. The only difference between this and a cholesteatoma is the absence of accumulation of epidermic squamae. The stratified squamous epithelium is classed as self-cleaning. Zechner [260] thinks that skin growth is more rapid at the centre of the pocket than at the circumference – the keratin layer migrates outwards, leaving the pocket free. Without wishing to anticipate the chapter on pathogenesis, it is obvious that the Eustachian tube and the inflammatory adhesion play an important part in the pathological process. It must, however, be distinguished from fibroadhesive otitis, in which a considerable, indeed very thick, fibroinflammatory layer is also present between the tympanic membrane and the mucosa, the epithelium of which is destroyed. This is not an artificial distinction. In fibroadhesive otitis, the cleavage can easily be made in the fibroinflammatory tissue – the problem is in getting rid of the inflamed appearance and obtaining a thin, normal mucosa. With the fixed retraction pocket, the difficulty lies in dissecting the epidermis, for any fragment left in the tympanic cavity is bound to develop into a cholesteatoma.

The Most Common Type of Fixed Retraction Pocket Is Posterior

There may be any intermediate stage between a pocket which can be partially elevated posteriorly and a complete epithelialization of the

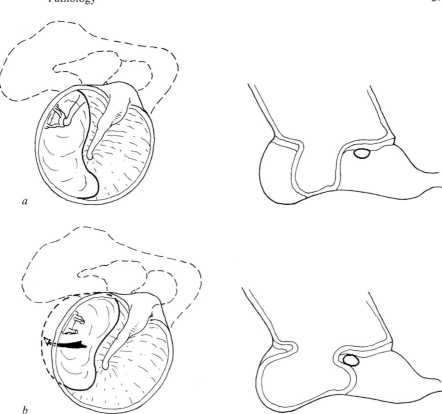

Fig. 13. Fixed retraction pocket in the posterior half of the tympanic cavity. *a* Pocket not affecting the posterior part of the mesotympanum. It is only fixed to the promontary. *b* Pocket adhering to the posterior part of the mesotympanum, destroying the short process of the incus and the superstructure of the stapes, and invading the three recesses of the posterior mesotympanum. Dissection is extremely difficult.

retrotympanum. In the first case, the pocket is fixed to the promontory and the edge of the round window, but is free posteriorly, separated from the back of the facial recess and the sinus tympani by some slightly inflammatory tissue which is none other than the mucosa of the medial surface of the tympanic membrane (fig. 13a). Sometimes there is a bed of granulation tissue or of polyps which may be inflamed and edematous in varying degrees. In such cases, dissection is rela-

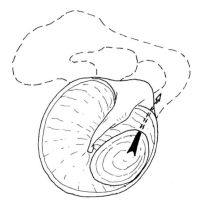

Fig. 14. Anterior fixed retraction pocket. Extending towards the Eustachian tube and the anterior attic.

tively easy. This granulation tissue often forms when it reaches the posterior sulcus, a small polypous protuberance in the shape of a truncated cone, which Sade [186, 187) has called a 'herodion'.

The difficulty is greatest, however, when the retrotympanum is epithelialized to a large extent. The epidermis adheres to the head of the stapes, the remaining parts of the incus, and the pyramidal process. It may extend downwards into the oval window, destroying the stapes or, even worse, covering it and its tendon. There is epithelialization of the three recesses of the retrotympanum, of which the sinus tympani presents the greatest difficulty (fig. 13b). Dissection of this type of epithelialization is extremely difficult, since the epithelium seems to adhere directly to the bone, with no appreciable plane of cleavage in connective tissue. Generally the pocket develops superiorly, posteriorly to the inferior process of the incus which is often destroyed, or anteriorly between the stapes and the tensor tympani tendon. In this cul-de-sac which goes beyond the diaphragm between the attic and the tympanic cavity, the desquamation will turn into a cholesteatoma if there is the slightest infection. In some cases very large cholesteatomas indeed may form from such posterior retraction pockets. In intermediate cases it may be difficult to draw a distinction between these retraction

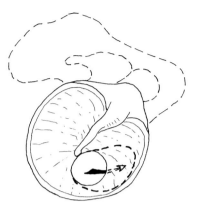

Fig. 15. Pouch-shaped fixed retraction pocket from a central perforation. Such cases are very rare. They may develop into cholesteatoma of the tympanic cavity.

pockets and true cholesteatomas. Very often, only exploratory surgery can determine the exact extent of the epithelial invasion, as radiology is often not sufficient.

Anterior Retraction Pockets Are Rarer

Such pockets generally develop from an anterior or kidney-shaped depression of the tympanic membrane. The pocket spreads towards the Eustachian tube and, as in the previous case, has a tendency to develop superiorly into the attic, but in this case anteriorly to the head of the malleus (fig. 14). Here again, desquamation, sometimes accelerated by infection, may form a cholesteatoma which varies from a limited to a very large one. It passed beneath the anterior tympanomalleolar ligament, and anteriorly to the tensor tympani tendon.

Retraction Pockets from Small Central Depression Are Exceptional

This pouch of skin extends medially from the tympanic membrane and adheres to a greater or lesser extent to the mucosa of the promontory. The bottom of the pouch may reach the orifice of the Eustachian tube and become invaginated in it to a greater or lesser degree. This

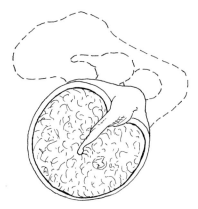

Fig. 16. Complete epithelialization of the bottom of the tympanic cavity. This is generally accompanied by the destruction of the incus and the stapes. Stapes fixation is not rare. In explaining this condition, it is difficult to determine the share of responsibility held by retraction from tubal insufficiency, and atrophic myringitis. Long-term prognosis for a reconstructed tympanic membrane is doubtful.

will be revealed during microscope examination, in the absence of which it might not be recognized and might be taken for an ordinary central perforation. It may develop into a cholesteatoma of the mesotympanum (fig. 15).

Epithelialization of the Medial Wall of the
Tympanic Cavity is Rarer

This may be taken for an atrophied tympanic membrane adhering to the promontary. The only way of distinguishing between the two is by insufflation which will partially elevate such a membrane. Some surgeons suggest that pure nitrous oxide should be inhaled for a few minutes, under surgical surveillance, in order to test this ability to be elevated. Medial to the sulcus and protruding remnants of the annulus, the skin lines the orifice of the Eustachian tube, and then the hypotympanum, and finally the region of the windows, becoming invaginated more or less beneath the edge of the lateral attic wall. It is a process of retraction and extremely fine adhesion, with no fibrous process, but with an attenuation of the fibrous layer of the tympanic membrane through atrophic myringitis (fig. 16). This may be called adhesive otitis.

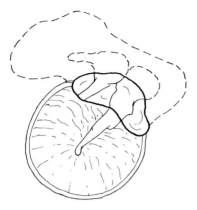

Fig. 17. Fixed attic retraction pocket. Here the attic wall is partially eroded and the pocket is lining the surface of the malleus and incus.

Retraction Pocket Fixed in the Attic

Such a condition is certainly even less stable than those we have just considered. There is often a slight retraction of the pars flaccida which moulds itself to the neck of the malleus, without the continuity of the epithelium disappearing from view under microscope examination. This is a picture which should alert the surgeon to the dysfunction of the Eustachian tube. In other cases the picture is much more clearly pathological, since the outer attic wall is partially eroded; but this erosion also makes it possible to inspect the whole of the surface of the pocket, which has no deep invagination (fig. 17). The situation is quite different when the pocket passes between the head of the malleus and the body of the incus on the one side and the outer attic wall on the other side. Here it is soon lost from sight and it is difficult to determine whether it stops a few millimetres beyond the free edge of the attic wall or whether it extends deeper into the attic. In some cases, because of limited bone erosion, it is possible, by inclining the patient's head and the microscope, to see that the retraction pocket passes over the body of the incus and the head of the malleus to line the medial and superior walls of the attic. When operating on such cases, it is rare not to find a lobe of cholesteatoma on a point of entering either the aditus or the

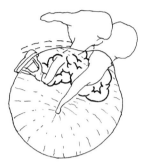

Fig. 18. Intact tympanic membrane cholesteatoma in the tympanic cavity. It takes the shape of a mass, sometimes surrounded by cholesterol granuloma situated inferiorly to the cochleariform process.

facial recess on the one hand, or extending towards the floor of the anterior attic or the region above the Eustachian tube on the other hand. These attic retraction pockets are particularly unstable and are quickly transformed into cholesteatomas if infection is present, whether the infection arrives through the Eustachian tube or through the meatus when bathing.

Intact Tympanic Membrane Cholesteatoma

These may be intrapetrous, particularly around the apex or the geniculate ganglion, or below the labyrinth. They are classified as primary cholesteatomas and will thus not be described here, even though they sometimes become apparent through conductive deafness as do intact tympanic membrane cholesteatomas of the middle ear [165]. We shall only describe intact tympanic membrane cholesteatomas of the middle ear here. They are not very common – 3.7% of 1,024 cases of cholesteatoma of the middle ear in the series of House and Sheehy [108] and 2% in the series of two of the present authors, one of which included 1071 cases, the other 699. The first seems to have been described in 1953 by House. An extensive survey of the literature in

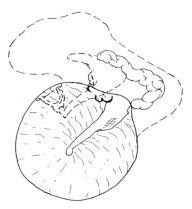

Fig. 19. Intact tympanic membrane cholesteatoma located in the medial attic. There may be a cholesterol granuloma in the mastoid. Damage to the ossicular chain may be extensive.

English has been made by Curtis [48] who collates 48 cases, reaching conclusions which are quite similar to those of one of the present authors in his series of 14 cases [40]. These cholesteatomas may be localized in the mesotympanum. They are more commonly found in children, usually in the anterosuperior region, and take the form of a pearl with a diameter of 2–6 mm. They adhere to the medial wall near the cochleariform process, and never extend higher than the facial nerve (fig. 18). They may extend to below the round window. In some cases, the pearl is surrounded by granulation tissue and cholesterol granuloma. In other cases, the cholesteatoma is situated in the posterosuperior part of the mesotympanum, and in these cases is very often accompanied by the destruction of the long process of the incus and the superstructure of the stapes. These locations seem to be commoner in older patients.

An equal number of closed tympanic cholesteatomas involve the attic (fig. 19) and usually also extend to the mesotympanum. They may be very limited, simple cholesteatoma pearls on the medial superior walls of the medial attic, accompanied by subacute lesions of the cholesterol granuloma type in the mastoid. In other cases, the lesions are much more extensive and the cholesteatoma destroys the superstructure of the stapes and the long process of the incus. Sometimes the

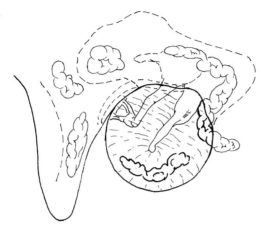

Fig. 20. Diffuse intact tympanic membrane cholesteatoma, combining cholesterol granuloma with stretches of epidermosis in the attic, mastoid and tympanic cavity.

whole of both the mesotympanum and the attic is invaded. It is interesting to point out that most of these cholesteatomas are situated on the medial attic wall. There may however be cases in the lateral attic, near a modified but still continuous pars flaccida. Finally, some intact tympanic membrane cholesteatomas extend not only to the attic and the mesotympanum but also to the mastoid. One of the present authors has observed a diffuse cholesteatoma in which cholesterol granuloma and epidermosis were mixed in the mesotympanum (fig. 20). Two of Derlacki's [54] cases showed pearls which were separated from the main mass. Goodhill [97] reports a case of a multilocular cholesteatoma of the temporal bone. It is interesting to point out that in the series of 37 cases reported by House and Sheehy [108], 50% of the intact tympanic membrane cholesteatomas were in patients under 20 years of age. Most had a developed mastoid. There may be complications – Curtis [48] mentions 2 cases of facial palsy, and House and Sheehy [108] mention a labyrinthine fistula. We may include intratympanic cholesteatomas [216, 225] with these intact tympanic membrane cholesteatomas. These are pearls set into the fibrous layer, but which may be predominantly medial or lateral. The pearl may be accompanied, as one of the present authors has observed, by a cholesterol granuloma developing in a highly sclerotic mastoid. Finally, there are three reported cases of cholesteatomas whose structure is dermoid rather than epithelial. Howie [cf. 108] reports a 4-mm dermoid cyst, of reddish colour, with hair follicles in the hypotympanum of a 29-year-old patient. Peron und Schuknecht [162] report a case of a dermoid cyst found in the attic and tympanic cavity of both ears, in an autopsy on a 20-year-old patient. These cysts, lined with keratinized epithelium, also contained epithelium with glandular hair cells, mucous glands, sebaceous glands and salivary glands.

Cholesteatoma of the External Auditory Meatus

Keratosis obturans (especially common in cases of Mounier-Kuhn's syndrome and Kartagener's syndrome) will in the long term give an oval shape to the meatus by eroding its bony walls which are covered by smooth skin, with no roughness at all. The mechanism is certainly the same as for bony erosion around a cholesteatoma. The appearance of the meatus may be greatly changed – the annulus seems to stand out, the outer attic wall may be thinner, almost nonexistent, or replaced by a mere membrance of skin which does not penetrate into the attic but resembles an enlargement of the pars flaccida; the relationship with the chorda tympani or even the facial nerve are changed; the skin may seem to cling closely to the chorda tympani or even the facial nerve. This is not, however, a true cholesteatoma of the meatus. With Mayer and Altman [cf. 166], we prefer to confine the use of the term 'cholesteatoma of the external auditory meatus' to invasions of epithelial tissue into the middle ear from a localized zone of periostitis of the meatus. Piepergerdes [166] et al. report observations of three such lesions which penetrated the floor of the meatus laterally to the annulus. In two cases the pathology was relatively limited. In one case the cholesteatoma sac exposed the third portion of the facial nerve over 1 cm and occupied the tip of the mastoid – the rest of the middle ear was healthy. Fifteen other cases have been reported in the literature on the subject. Symptoms include both pain and suppuration and the differential diagnosis is of course to be made with cancer of the external auditory meatus, diabetic osteitis and the rare benign osteitis confined to the meatus. Some cholesteatomas occupy both the external auditory meatus and the middle ear, almost reaching the opening of the meatus often exposing the third portion of the facial nerve which may be free on the medial side of the cholesteatoma. In other cases the cholesteatoma erodes and penetrates the inner ear; in this case the genu and second portion of the facial nerve are surrounded by the cholesteatoma. Surgery of such lesions must be very careful in order to avoid damage to the facial nerve. From the point of view of pathogenesis, it is difficult to say whether the starting-point of the cholesteatoma was in the meatus or the middle ear.

Finally, one of the present authors has encountered, in a 2-year-old child, a cholesteatoma situated behind the skin of the external auditory meatus, causing a stenosis of the meatus. The sac had eroded an unobstrusive hollow in the bone of the posterior canal wall and could be dissected as far as its pedicle which, curiously enough, appeared to lead towards the area of the pars flaccida. It is also possible to find a small cholesteatoma of the floor of the meatus at the superior end of a fistula of the first branchial cleft.

Extension of Cholesteatomas of the Middle Ear to within the Petrous Bone

Extension of cholesteatomas of the middle ear to within the petrous bone generally follows the preformed cell tracts [35, 71, 73, 142, 150, 172].

Anterior extension above the labyrinth follows the anterior supralabyrinthine tract above the second portion of the facial nerve and the geniculate ganglion, passing anteriorly to the ampulla of the superior semicircular canal and developing between the vestibule laterally, the internal auditory meatus medially and the cochlea inferiorly. These various organs may be exposed or opened. In some cases the endosteum of the vestibule remains intact, in others it is opened.

A retrolabyrinthine extension follows the retrolabyrinthine cell tract behind the superior semicircular canal and above the posterior semicircular canal. The cholesteatoma then turns medially and may reach, from behind, this same zone situated between the internal auditory meatus medially and the vestibule laterally, going on to develop in the area of the first portion of the facial nerve.

A translabyrinthine extension may reach this same zone by following the translabyrinthine cell tract, the subarcuate artery and the vestige of the petromastoid canal.

A infralabyrinthine extension, finally, will follow the posterior sublabyrinthine tract, the size of which will depend on the height of the jugular bulb. If the bulb is very high, it closes the posteroinferior angle of the tympanic cavity. If, on the other hand, the jugular bulb is not prominent (this is the case for 30% of temporal bones according to Girard [92]), the groups of cells starting from the hypotympanum and the retrofacial and occipitojugular region come together beneath the labyrinth to form a large infralabyrinthine cell tract which goes on towards the tip of the petrous bone, passing medially to the third portion of the facial nerve, beneath the labyrinth and beneath the internal auditory meatus. The cholesteatoma often enters these different zones, especially the posterior weak point of the tympanic cavity where it enters the posterior cells of the hypotympanum, medially to the facial nerve, forming a mass extending towards the cell tract between the facial nerve and the sigmoid sinus. It may also develop anteriorly in the area of the internal carotid artery, in the cells of the anterior hypotympanum, and may extend to the floor of the Eustachian tube. The cholesteatoma may of course be larger and extend medially, forming a single, or multilobed, mass reaching the tip of the petrous bone. During its progress it will push the jugular bulb posteriorly, and anteriorly it pushes back or exposes the internal carotid artery; further on, it exposes the cochlea and then the internal auditory meatus. These extensions of course raise the question of pathogenesis. In a fair number of cases, it is clear, from the fact that there has been suppuration over a long period, and that there is a perforation of varying size, of the tympanic membrane, and from the respective size of the lesions which are mainly in the middle ear, that on ordinary cholesteatoma of the middle ear has extended to the petrous bone. In other cases, the cholesteatoma seems to have extended into the middle ear, into the medial attic or the translabyrinthine cell tract, while its main mass is located in the petrous bone. This is certainly a primary, congenital cholesteatoma. The situation may be even more confused by the fact that a cholesteatoma of the petrous bone may have an indirect effect on the middle ear by causing stenosis of the Eustachian tube, and thus mucous otitis, a retraction pocket and a perforation of the tympanic membrane.

Microscopic Appearances

The term 'cholesteatoma' was first used by Johannes Muller in 1838. He described its layered structure and its capsule of epithelium.

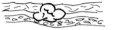

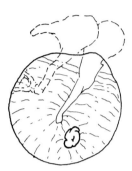

Fig. 21. Intratympanic cholesteatoma. The cholesteatoma pearl is set into the fibrous layer but may be predominantly medial or lateral. This pearl may be accompanied by inflammatory lesions such as a mastoid cholesterol granuloma (observed by one of the present authors).

The term 'epidermoid cyst of the ear' or 'keratoma' [197] would be more accurate since it describes the real role played by the keratinized epithelium. A cholesteatoma is in fact an accumulation of desquamated keratin in the middle ear, surrounded by a matrix composed of basal cells and the stratum malpighii of the squamous keratinized epithelium.

Composition of a Cholesteatoma

A cholesteatoma is usually formed of layers of epithelium, which may be thick or thin, arranged like the layers of an onion, deteriorating nearer the centre where they become amorphous. This is the dry cholesteatoma. When the cholesteatoma is open and infected, the central mass is soft and suppurating – only the matrix can be identified. In such cases especially, examination of a cross section reveals bands of connective tissue rich in fatty granulations produced by the disintegration of inflamed cells, intermingled with remnants of epithelium. These apparently contradictory observations can be explained by the degree of inflammatory reaction in the chorion, the rupture of the basal cell layer or the papillary structure of the cholesteatoma.

Cholesteatoma Matrix

The matrix is the starting-point of the cholesteatoma and determines how far it will extend. It is composed of keratinized or even
hyperkeratosic Malpighian epithelium resting on connective chorion
(fig. 21).

Epithelial Layer

This is thinner than in the skin and contains no papillae or dermal appendages. It consists of the four epithelial layers which represent the
differentiation of the basal cell pushed towards the surface (fig. 22).

The stratum germinativum is made up of small prismatic cells with
large basophilic nuclei, arranged in a layer. As they multiply the epithelial cells are renewed, which explains the occurrence of mitosis.

The stratum spinosum is composed of larger polyhedric cells with
central nuclei. These are joined by points between the cells, which
gives an appearance of spiny cells under the microscope. This layer
comprises only 2 or 3 strata of cells.

The stratum granulosum is made up of a single layer of lozenge-
shaped cells, flattened parallel to the surface. Their nuclei are beginning to degenerate and their cytoplasm to become saturated with
dense keratohyalin granulations.

The stratum corneum includes several layers of acidophilic, flattened completely keratinized cells, in which the pyknotic nucleus disappears and the plasma membrane thickens. These cells, which have
reached complete maturity, degenerate and desquamate. These lamellae of keratin, which are particularly important in the cholesteatoma,
form the contents of the sac. These layers are sometimes considerably
modified. Sometimes only the keratinized layer is visible, sometimes
both the keratinized and granular layers can be seen.

The characteristics of the ultrastructure of the different cell layers
are identical to those of the epidermis. The cells, or keratinocytes, are
linked by desmosomes and contain in their cytoplasm tonofibrils
which join to the desmosomes and come together in thick bunches in
the stratum spinosum. In the stratum granulosum there are, in the cytoplasm, dense masses formed by the densification of fibrillar structures, and which are made of keratohyalin. In the stratum corneum,
these granules come together and fill the cytoplasm, while the pyknotic
nuclei disappear. Bremond et al. [27], to whom we are indebted, em-

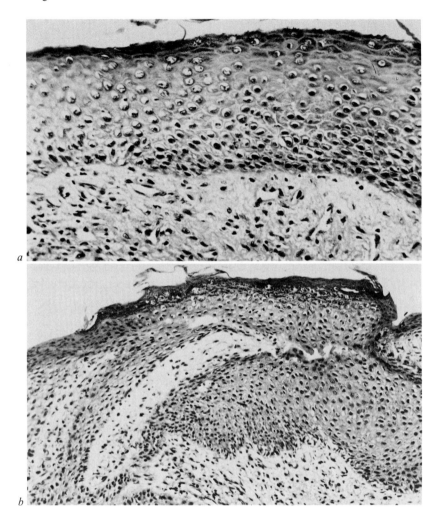

Fig. 22. Cholesteatoma matrix (H11 1868): a highly inflamed chorion is covered with Malpighian epithelium composed of a granular layer and keratinized squames. On the left *(a)* parakeratosis is beginning. This covering comes direct on a layer of cylindrical epithelium. *a* 200× – final enlargement 640. *b* 63× – final enlargement 200. (Photograph provided by Prof. Couderc, Histology Laboratory of Grenoble University Hospital).

phasize the presence of two particular types of cell, which are also present in skin coverings but have only been described in cholesteatomas.

Langerhans' cells are found in the stratum spinosum between the keratinocytes, to which they are not joined in any way, and from which they are separated by an open space. Their general appearance is clear, their nuclei are irregularly shaped and marked by many invaginations. Their cytoplasm, which lacks tonofibrils, contains large mitochondria, and especially a characteristic organella in the shape of a small vesicle, extended by a rod 400 Å in diameter and between 0.1 and 0.3 μm long. These are more common in the cholesteatoma matrix than in the skin of a normal tympanic membrane.

Merkel's cells are clear cells located in the stratum germinativum and linked by desmosomes to neighbouring keratinocytes. Their large, lobed, twisted nuclei resemble those of Langerhans' cells, but they are distinguishable by their smaller size, a more lobular shape and the absence of the characteristic organellas. Their clear cytoplasm contains a large number of mitochondria and, especially, small, dense, rounded, very osmiophilic granules.

These same authors stress that the presence of these cells, which are not present in normal middle ear mucosa, seems to argue in favor of the migration theory. They also emphasize the fact that the skin of the floor of the external auditory meatus has the same histological and ultrastructural appearence as the cholesteatoma.

Basement Membrane

A hyaline basement membrane separates the stratum germinativum from the connective chorion. It may be smooth or undulating, with depressions caused by expansion of cells in the basal cell layer. Its thickness is comparable to that of the epidermic basement membrane. It may be papillary, in which case each papilla penetrates, to a varying degree, into the contents of the cholesteatoma. The connective basis of the papilla appears in the epithelial lamellae in transverse sections, which explains the presence of connective tissue within the cholesteatoma.

This basement membrane may disappear, and the epithelium may lie directly on the connective layer, causing large macrophages to appear. It is important to stress that in this way the keratinized epithelium may migrate into the thickness of the middle ear mucosa.

Examination of the ultrastructure of the basement membrane shows that it is attached to the germinative cells by hemidesmosomes, and fixed to the chorion by reticulinic fibrils. It is generally admitted than the basement membrane is formed from the epithelial cells which lie on it and not from connective tissue. The epithelial cells have the same antigenic properties and the same staining characteristics as the lamina basalis.

Connective Chorion

The connective layer is of variable thickness, depending on how inflamed it is. It may be extremely thin, in which case the epithelium appears to lie directly on the bone, or on the contrary extremely thick, in which case it is easier to detach. This chorion is in close contact with the underlying bone. It is rich in mucopolysaccharides and mucoproteins.

Unterlying the basal cells, reticulin fibrils and elastic fibres of varying dimensions are to be found; they form a loose network penetrating the vascular canals and the areas of erosion of the underlying bone. Only the reticulin fibrils appear to be attached to the bone. Layers of collagen are found nearer the bone. The arrangement of these is less dense than in normal skin. They continue from the adventitia of the bone vessels and sometimes extend to the surface perpendicularly to the epithelial basement layer. They may also, particularly in this area, become fragmented, disintegrate and lose their orientation. The most common cells in the subepithelial space are fibroblasts, which are generally immature. The are close to the underlying bone and appear active when the cholesteatoma grows. These fibroblasts produce large quantities of precollagenic fibres.

As we have seen, this connective tissue is subject, to a variable degree, to lymphocytic and plasmocytic infiltration. This inflammation may lead to an inflammatory granuloma, and the chorion may be transformed, totally or in patches, into granulation tissue which may be fibrous in varying degrees. This tissue is infiltrated by inflammatory cells, which are basically of the lymphoplasmocytic type. Crystals of cholesterol and hemosiderinic pigments are deposited. There are macrophages containing phagosomes which may by empty or filled with lipidic vacuoles and hemosiderin. Many vessels, and degraded red blood cells which provide pigments, are also found. Finally, small mucous glands may be found.

Migration of Epithelium and the Mucosa

In some cases it is possible to examine the boundary between the matrix and the mucosa [125, 126]. Here, the mucosa is always inflamed. The forward limit of the matrix includes highly papillary basal cells and an intricate system of linkage. In most cases, the epithelial cells infiltrate the chorion of the inflamed mucosa. This conflict between the skin and the mucosa is resolved by a system of contact guidance by the linking fibres between the advanting front of the epithelial matrix and the inflamed mucous tissue.

Reactions Around the Cholesteatoma

In the Bone

The reaction of the temporal bone to a cholesteatoma has been compared to osteomyelitis of long bones. The destruction of the bone is associated with reconstruction and sclerosis. In fact, osteomyelitis is a term which can only be used in connection with bones possessing a medulla, whereas in the vast majority of cases we are concerned with an osteitis of the septa between the air cells and of the cortex. These lesions are the same as those found in other forms of progressive chronic otitis media. It is nonetheless certain that destruction of the bone is more common and more widespread when a cholesteatoma is present [189, 240]. Kanedo et al. [119] have calculated this frequency by comparing a series of 100 petrous bones with cholesteatoma and another series of 100 petrous bones with chronic otitis media but no cholesteatoma. In the first case, the bone was destroyed in 80% of the cases while bone destruction was only found in 25% of the cases without cholesteatoma.

A distinction must however be made between two aspects of these changes due to the presence of a cholesteatoma – the direct influence of contact with the cholesteatoma itself and the indirect influence which is linked to the presence of a cholesteatoma at a certain distance. In the former case, a layer of connective tissue, even if it is extremely thin, may still seem to be present beneath the epithelium. Sade and Halevy [190], then Sade and Berco [189], have observed, between the bone and the epithelium, connective tissue which is generally severely inflamed. Lim et al. [125], using an electron microscope, have

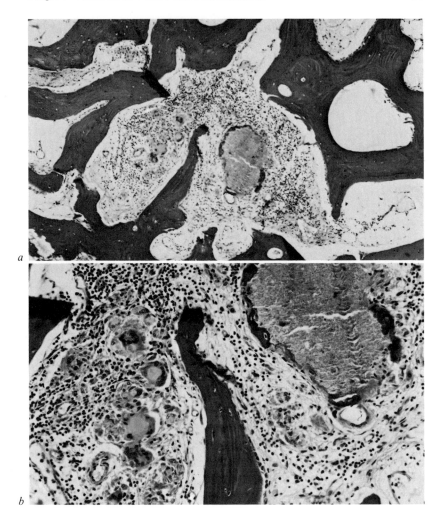

Fig. 23. Osteitis of the mastoid tip (G46466C). Inflammatory granuloma with giant cells near a necrobiotic sequestrum. *a* 63 × – final enlargement 200. *b* 200 × – final enlargement 640. (Photographs provided by Prof. Couderc, Histology Laboratory of Grenoble University Hospital.)

also observed that there is always an extremely thin layer of connective tissue beneath the epithelium of the cholesteatoma, although examination with an optical microscope may seem to show the cholesteatoma in direct contact with the bone. This connective tissue contains very few collagen fibres. Crystalline structures comparable to those found in osteoclasts may be found.

Kaneko et al. [119] stress that bone destruction is frequent around zones where the matrix is broken, allowing keratin to penetrate into the connective tissue where it causes a tissue reaction consisting of cell infiltration, giant cells and cholesterol crystals. Tos [240] and Abramson and Chen-Chung [5] had also observed that bone destruction was found mainly around the cholesteatoma sac. Reactions of the bone which are indirectly linked to the presence of the cholesteatoma are the same as those found in all cases of chronic otitis media, particularly in the mastoid. Both direct and indirect reactions are found in the bony canal, the ossicles and the labyrinth.

Mastoid

The mastoid may be healthy if there is no infection within the cholesteatoma, and if it does not hinder the aeration of the mastoid cells. If there is infection, osteitis, comparable to the osteitis found in chronic otitis media without cholesteatoma, will develop. It may progress rapidly through a mastoid which is still highly pneumatized, especially in a child (fig. 23). In the sclerotic eburnated zones, on the other hand, the bone is thick, the Haversian canals are empty or fibrous, and the bone is richly impregnated with calcium salts. In some cases, the lines of bone apposition are clearly visible [82], with dark blue colouring, in a glacier-like arrangement, with an associated pagetoid appearance of more irregular lines, like a mosaic. It is also interesting to note that Friedman [82] stresses that new bone formation is a fundamental process in otitis media, forming secondary sclerotic bone – he has shown experimentally, following Opheim [cf.82], that a such transformation is possible. Like Ruedi [181], Tumarkin [cf.17, 128] and Ojala and Palva [cf.82], he thinks that this sclerosis of the mastoid is the result and not the cause of chronic suppuration. If the cholesteatoma obstructs the aeration of the mastoid, a cholesterol granuloma will appear in varying locations. Depending on the location of the obstruction, it may fill just the mastoid cells, or even the antrum, or part of the attic. It may form a thick, lardaceous layer around the matrix. The

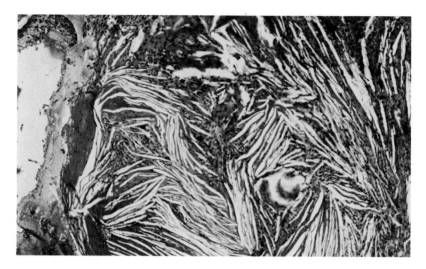

Fig. 24. Extremely typical cholesterol granuloma in the antrum, with a large number of needle-shaped cholesterol crystals (G51758A). 63× – final enlargement 200. (Photograph provided by Prof. Couderc, Pathology Laboratory of Grenoble University Hospital.)

mastoid takes on a sappy yellowish appearance. Sometimes there are lesions very similar to those of a mucous otitis – there is a mucous effusion, sometimes blackish, in large cells lined with a thick mucosa.

This cholesterol granuloma is formed from fibrous granulation tissue, in which a large number of cholesterol crystals, surrounded by giant cells with foreign bodies, are found (fig. 24). This granulation tissue often shows signs of recent bleeding, such as the presence of hemosiderin. Linthicum's [128] experiments, demonstrating the formation of cholesterol granuloma by the blocking of ventilation, should also be noted.

Bony Canal

This is sometimes extensive destruction of the bony canal by the cholesteatoma, carrying out a spontaneous atticoantrotomy, which may cure the lesions, or which may be insufficient to exteriorize a large

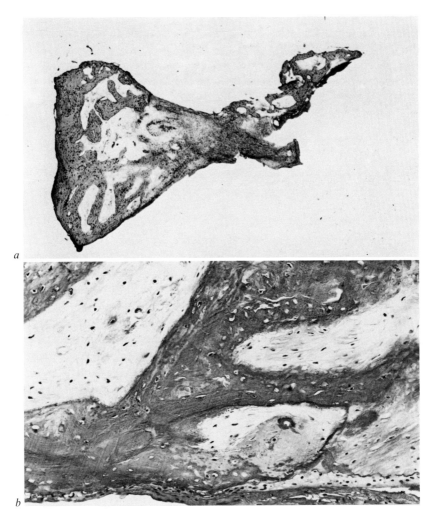

Fig. 25. Erosion of the incus, which has been reduced to a few fibrous remnants and a stump – bony tissue whose cavities have been rearranged by noninflammatory fibrosis associated with dystrophic lesions of the bony lamellae. Powdery calcification. *a* 25 × – final enlargement 40. *b* 200 × – final enlargement 320. (Photograph provided by Prof. Couderc, Pathology Laboratory of Grenoble University Hospital.)

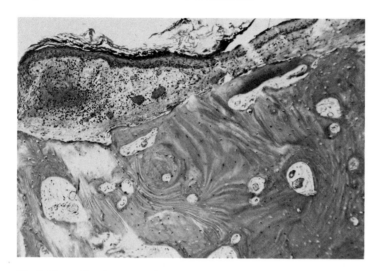

Fig. 26. Incus lined at one point by a cholesteatoma (H1533). 63 × – final enlargement 200. (Photograph provided by Prof. Couderc, Pathology Laboratory of Grenoble University Hospital.)

cholesteatoma. Partial destruction of the outer attic wall in very common, the actual degree of destruction being variable. This is one of the difficulties met with in the closed technique, and it may cause the surgeon to change to an open technique. It is rare to find a Gelle's fistula in the posterior part of the external auditory meatus. It is sometimes found under the canal skin or during the dissection of cholesteatoma using a transmastoid approach.

Ossicles

Sade and Halevy [190] have compared the ossicles of 25 patients suffering from cholesteatoma with those of 75 patients suffering from chronic otitis media without cholesteatoma. In the former group there was destruction of the ossicles in 95% of the cases, most frequently affecting the incus (95%), and then, with equal frequency, the malleus and the stapes (33%). Destruction of the ossicles was half as common in the group with no cholesteatoma – 42%. These points are frequently confirmed by observations.

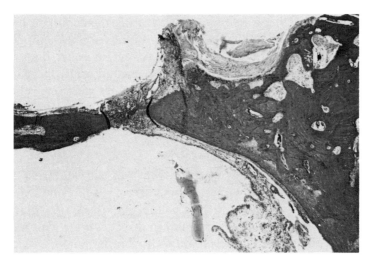

Fig. 27. Erosion of the long process of the incus, caused by osteitis accompanying a cholesteatoma (H1533). 15× – final enlargement 50. (Photograph provided by Prof. Couderc, Pathology Laboratory of Grenoble University Hospital.)

The most commonly destroyed area of the incus is the long process. The particularly fragile nature of its afferent vessels may be mentioned. The lenticular process often remains, attached to the head of the stapes. The body of the incus may be covered with large eroded areas over its medial or lateral surface. The short process may be destroyed. In some cases, only a 'ghost' incus remains (fig. 25). In other cases, finally, only the body of the incus is destroyed, leaving a long process closely attached to the stapes while the incus and the malleus have been destroyed (fig. 26, 27). The head of the malleus is destroyed in isolation in cholesteatomas of the anterior attic. It may be completely destroyed while the incus remains intact, although this is rare. The malleus handle may be eroded, especially in cases of epithelialization of the tympanic cavity. Finally, the stapes may be affected in a number of different ways. It may be totally destroyed, with the epithelium adhering closely to the footplate. In other cases, a layer of granulation tissue or a mucous membrane separates the skin from the footplate, making it easier to dissect. Sometimes a stump, or even a whole crus remains, involving a real risk of fracturing the footplate during dissection, since the crus will act as a lever if it has not been noticed in the cholesteatomatous tissue. The crura may remain intact, but practically devitalized, and will not be found if a second stage operation is performed. A particularly difficult situation is met with when the superstructure remains but without a stapes head. It is often situated medially to the facial ridge, and the ossicular chain is extremely difficult to reconstruct.

This destruction of the ossicles has been studied in particular by Sade and Berco [189] on 39 ossicles from patients suffering from chronic otitis media whith cholesteatoma. The area of bone which is destroyed is always covered either by connective tissue or by granulation tissue – no epithelium is ever found in direct contact with the destroyed area. 20% of the ossicles showed an inflammatory reaction deep in the bone. We have made the same observations on our own samples – destruction is quicker than in the mastoid because of the smaller size and poor blood supply of the ossicles. There are three stages in the destruction: (1) myelitis, which is a congestive stage; (2) osteolytic necrosis, which is the replacement of the bone by granulation tissue from the surface or rather from the medullary spaces, and (3) eburnating osteosis which leads to the formation of a compact bone, while the granulation tissue is transformed into fibrous tissue. Samples of partially eroded ossicles reveal bony lamellae, irregularly impregnated with calcium. Their outline is very irregular and undergoing a process of necrosis from contact with granulocytes, lymphocytes and plasmocytes in an inflammatory granuloma held by fibrous lamellae or collagens. All the medullary spaces are not affected. Some areas may be completely normal next to spaces filled with small abscesses. Penetration of a cholesteatoma into the ossicles is problematical, though rare. Sade [184] observed it on six occasions out of 50 ossicles. One of the present authors has met with it twice in a series of 100 cases. We never transpose an ossicle which has been in contact with a cholesteatoma. A cholesteatoma may not merely destroy the ossicular chain, it may fix it through the bone reconstruction: fixation of the malleus and/or the incus, and more rarely stapedovestibular ankylosis. It is impossible to say whether this is a tympanosclerosis which has become secondarily ossified, a disorganized production of bone to reconstruct a zone of osteitis, or, in the footplate, osteoarthritis as Goodhill [98] suggested, or an associated otosclerosis.

Labyrinth

The main data in this section have been taken from previous works of one of the present authors [251, 253]. 120 fistulae of the lateral semicircular canal, representing 11% of the cholesteatoma operations performed by this author, were collated. The lateral semicircular canal is not the only location since, in the same series, the author observed 3 fistulae of the superior semicircular canal, 3 on the posterior canal, 3 on the promontary, 2 at the oval window and the footplate, and 1 on the anterior part of the cochlea (a total of 6 cochlear fistulae). These fistulae may be found on old mastoid cavities (12% of cases) demonstrating that the destruction of the labyrinthine capsule by a cholesteatoma is not simply caused by mechanical pressure. A fistula on the lateral semicircular canal is situated on the middle of the convexity, or slightly lateral to it, in 50% of cases. It is definitely posterior to the top of the convexity in 26% of cases while an anterior location is only found in 8%. The convexity was totally destroyed in 16% of the cases.

Using Gacek's [83] classification, the author distinguishes between precursor of fistula, large fistula and narrow fistula. A precursor of fistula is found in 7% of the cases, where a bluish line generally marks the dome of the convexity of the semicircular canal. Palpation is to be avoided. Large fistulae are generally over 2 mm long and at least 0.5 mm wide. The appearance of the edges varies according to the reaction around the matrix. They may be the seat of granulomatous lesions which are difficult to remove. When the matrix is easy to detach, the fistula takes on the appearance of a gently sloped 'valley'. The author recommends that the fistula should be illuminated with a green light from the microscope, and that the surgeon should check the continuity of the endosteum by gentle palpation of the footplate of the stapes. Sometimes the membranous canal may be reddish or vitrified. Narrow fistulae are usually less than 2 mm long. They are never more than 0.5 mm wide. The edges are often abrupt, and the endosteum is commonly intact. The cholesteatoma matrix forms a bridge over the edges, or shows a small finger-like depression at this point, where it can easily be detached.

The cholesteatoma accompanying the fistula is always large, reaching or going beyond the mastoid antrum in 90% of the cases. It is interesting to note, on the other hand, that this author observed only one fistula where there was no cholesteatoma. The facial canal was open or dehiscent in 35% of the cases. In 8 cases, facial palsy was observed at the same time as the fistula. There was also exposure of other important structures – the meninges in 22 cases, the lateral sinus in 3 cases and the internal carotid artery in 1 case. Furthermore, 1 extradural empyema, 3 cases of meningitis (1 of which was accompanied by a temporal abscess) and 1 cerebellar abscess were found at the same time as the fistula. We shall adopt the same histological and prognostic classification as Wayoff and Bremond [251].

Stage I – Precursor of fistula, bony shell relatively solid, excellent prognosis.

Stage II – Erosion of the bone complete with endosteum intact, functional prognosis generally very good.

Stage II – Fistula with destruction of the endosteum, but no intralabyrinthine lesions – these are generally narrow fistulae with abrupt edges.

Stage IV – The endosteum is obviously destroyed, and a distinction must be made between limited perilabyrinthitis, with apparent septation of the lumen of the canal, and absence of perilymph even when the oval window is palpated, and the rupture of the septa, with perilymph appearing during surgery, this being generally a sign of diffuse perilabyrinthitis. In this latter case the functional prognosis is very poor.

Stage V – The membranous canal is invaded by inflammatory elements, there is diffuse labyrinthitis. Such ears have usually been deaf for some time. We might add a *stage VI* – invasion of the labyrinth by the cholesteatoma, which is a case we have encountered on several occasions. The cholesteatoma passes into the vestibule which is widely opened above the facial nerve, and progresses, often at a distance, following the semicircular canals and, anteriorly, the cochlea. In other cases, the posterior labyrinth is partially or totally destroyed. Bumsted et al. [30], however, have reported the retention of subnormal hearing despite a subtotal destruction of the posterior labyrinth. These anomalies can no doubt be explained by septation. We have met with several observations of this type. In contrast with fistulae of the semicircular canals, and especially of the lateral canal, fistulae of the promontory have a very severe functional prognosis. Many authors, including Palva et al. [158] 2 cases, Ritter [176] 1 case, Abramson et al. [7] 3 cases, and Martin and Martin [141] 1 case, stress that sensorineural impairment is practically inevitable if an attempt is made to remove the epithelial sac of the cholesteatoma. Our experience confirms these observations entirely. The reason is given by Gacek [83] – the presence of a fistula on the wall of the cochlea exposes the endosteum around the spiral ligament, close to the stria vascularis which may be damaged by the removal of the epithelium. One of the present authors has observed 4 cochlear fistulae, 2 of which actually dissected the whole of the cochlea, with complete preoperative deafness, while the other 2 were more limited, and led to total postoperative deafness – in one case, 6 months after surgery. Martin and Martin [141], however, report an observation on a subtotal destruction of the anterior part of the cochlea, leaving some residual hearing.

In our series we have observed 142 fistulae of the lateral semicircular canal, and 3 cochlear fistulae, out of 1,856 cases of cholesteatoma (7.8%).

Facial Nerve

In quite a large number of cases, the facial nerve is naturally dehiscent above the oval window on its inferior slope or inferolateral half of its circumference. It may also be dehiscent near a cell or Sappey's fossa which may expose it in its third portion, either immediately at the genu, or lower. This is fairly rare as the facial nerve is normally situated in solid bone [44]. Around the second portion, the cholesteatoma may develop within the oval window niche and adhere to the nerve if it is already dehiscent, or help to expose it. In fact, around the second portion of the facial nerve, the cholesteatoma much more often exposes the anterior part of the second portion, immediately anterior to the lateral semicircular canal, above the cochleariform process. It is therefore necessary, when dissecting the medial wall of the attic, to locate the second portion of the facial nerve in order to avoid damaging it if it is exposed. Sometimes this exposure continues as far as the beginning of the second portion, favouring invasion of the supra-tubal recess. The surface of the lateral slope of the geniculate ganglion and the petrosal nerve may be exposed. In rare cases, the whole of the second portion of the facial nerve is exposed over threequarters of its circumference. Extreme care must be taken in detaching the matrix, and there is an obvious, though not inevitable, risk of postoperative paresis or even secondary paralysis.

The threat to the facial nerve is even greater when there is an intralabyrinthine cholesteatoma . In such cases the cholesteatoma completely surrounds the facial nerve which may even be lost within it. Total deafness, accompanying a large cholesteatoma, is a sign which should alert the surgeon to this situation, which requires him to locate the facial nerve in healthy bone, generally the third portion, in order to be able to dissect it step by step. The third portion of the facial nerve may be exposed near the lower part of the chorda tympani, by an extension of a cholesteatoma into the facial recess. Lower down, the facial nerve may be exposed on its medial surface by a cholesteatoma penetrating the posteroinferior weakpoint of the tympanic cavity and passing into the posterior infralabyrinthine cell tract. In a few exceptional cases, the third portion of the facial nerve may be completely exposed by the cholesteatoma which, in this event, embraces the exposed nerve from the ampulla of the posterior semicircular canal as far as the stylomastoid foramen. In such a situation it is of course necessary first to locate the genu and the second portion of the facial nerve to continue the dissection. In cases of extensions within the petrous bone, the first portion of the facial nerve may be completely exposed from the internal auditory meatus as far as the geniculate ganglion. Where there are supralabyrinthine extensions which open the internal auditory meatus on its superior surface, the nerve may be distended and frayed by the labyrinth, and the contents of the meatus may be lowered by the mass of the cholesteatoma. When the extensions are infralabyrinthine, on the other hand, it may be raised from the internal auditory meatus which is opened by its inferior surface. Great care must be taken when dissecting it. If the facial nerve is already clinically paralysed, it is often so fragile that it will inevitably rupture, making suturing or a graft necessary.

Meninges and the Lateral Sinus

We shall only mention direct lesions to the meninges and the lateral sinus here, reserving discussion of the infectious complications to the chapter on complications. The dura is rarely exposed over an extended area by a cholesteatoma. A thin film of bone, which may be mobile, remains in contact with the temporal or cerebellar meninges. This bony layer makes it easier to dissect the cholesteatoma matrix, which otherwise will adhere very closely to the dura itself, which may make the dissection very long and difficult, working in layers, encroaching on the dural tissue, with the risk of causing a breach.

Sometimes the external temporal dura mater is prolapsed and it may be necessary to raise it with a thin layer of bone in order to get at a deep recess which is situated higher. This may be necessary both in the open technique and in the closed technique. The surgeon must however be careful not to leave too large an area of dura exposed, remembering that all progressive meningoencephaloceles are due to a rupture of the dura mater. It is nonetheless wise to line the meninges with a sheet of periosteum whenever it is certain that a residual cholesteatoma is not being buried.

The lateral sinus is rarely in contact with the cholesteatoma. If it does adhere, dissection from its wall is extremely difficult, unless infection has opportunely created granulation tissue, making it possible to dissect the matrix.

Tympanic Cavity and the Eustachian Tube

The tympanic cavity of an ear affected by a cholesteatoma may be perfectly healthy in the mesotympanum and the hypotympanum. The cholesteatoma may reach no further than the inferior limit of the attic, even though it may have a very large posterior extension. In other cases, one or several lobes of cholesteatoma penetrate the mesotympanum from above downwards as we have seen. The tympanic cavity may also be partially occupied by an epithelialization, generally in the posterior part of the mesotympanum, and this may stop here or form a cholesteatoma which may be very large. We should like, very briefly, to stress here the inflammatory aspects ot the tympanic cavity and the Eustachian tube which may accompany the cholesteatoma, whether or not it affects this zone directly. In a considerable number of cases, the mucosa of the tympanic cavity is inflamed and oedematous. If the inflammation is more severe it may be filled by a seromucinous effusion. Sometimes the mucosa is so inflamed that it transforms the whole of the promontory and the hypotympanum into an extremely pathological granulation tissue, which must be removed, leaving the mucoperiosteum intact.

Finally, in a few cases, the inflammatory process in the tympanic cavity has died down over a period of many years, and has become modified into a thick layer of fibrocholesterol tissue, which may or may not include pockets of mucus, and which constitutes a fibroadhesive otitis. These accompanying lesions must not be ignored since, to a great extent, it is on them that the prognosis of a tympanoplasty will depend.

Histogenous Mechanisms Involved in
Destruction of Bone by Cholesteatoma

In order to explain the destructive capacities of cholesteatoma and its extension, two theories have been put forward: erosion by compression and enzymatic erosion.

Successful treatment by suction [145] or by marsupialization, leaving the cholesteatoma matrix intact [15], habe been put forward as arguments in favour of the theory of erosion by compression, caused by an accumulation of keratin lamellae in the matrix [181, 244]. However, long-term follow-up of these cavities quite often shows up a change, and we have pointed out that fistulae of the lateral semicircular canal may develop in mastoid cavities which appear to be stable.

Enzymatic erosion has been studied extensively during the last 10 years. Walsh et al. [249] thought enzymatic substances from the matrix or from the epithelial debris could destroy the bone. The histochemical work of Abramson and co-workers [3–6], Thomsen et al. [235] and Harris [103] suggests that the most important factor in bone destruction may be hydrolytic, lysosomal, or enzymatic, situated in the subepithelial granulation tissue. Abramson and Chen-Chung [4] have found a significant quantity of collagenase in a cholesteatoma and in the deep skin of the external auditory meatus. This collagenase activity is increased when granulation tissue is present. Bernstein et al. [18] have shown that there is, in cholesteatomatous material, a factor which stimulates demineralization of the bone, and suggest that a soluble cholesteatoma extract can produce calcium resorption, stimulate osteoclastic activity and inhibit bone formation. The factor in question could be an endoxin or lipotechoic acid [104], a prostaglandin [120] or a factor which activates osteoclasts [106].

Interaction between the cholesteatoma and the granulation tissue should not be discounted as certain histopathological findings suggest since superinfected granulation tissue is rich in enzymes and highly vascularized. Thomsen et al. [235] stress that the mechanism of bone destruction is the same in all cases of suppurative chronic otitis media whether or not a cholesteatoma is present – optical and electronic microscopy show that the superficial layer of the submucosa is dominated by inflammatory cells, fibrocytes and fibroblasts in a stroma of loose, collagen-type connective tissue. In the zones nearest the underlying eroded bone, the predominant type of cell is the histiocyte, found in a close relationship with a proliferating, active capillary network. This increased vascularization seems to be directly linked to the bone destruction.

Gantz and Maynard [88] sum up their work by stressing that both demineralization and collagen degradation are necessary for bone destruction to take place. Lysosomal acid phosphatase is found in large quantities in the cytoplasm of inflammatory mononuclear cells attached to the edges of zones of bone resorption. These cells are not osteoclasts. Phosphatase is more rarely found in fibroblasts in the inflammatory tissue, and it also exists in the extracellular environment. In the bone adjacent to the zone of resorption, the osteocytes also contain acid phosphatase. Collagenase is also found in the extracellular spaces surrounding the inflammatory mononuclear cells and the edge of the osteocytes.

Iatrogenic Cholesteatomas

Iatrogenic Cholesteatomas Caused by Inadequate Diagnosis

These are found after myringoplasties performed on perforations which appear simple but which in fact involve an undetected epithelialization of the tympanic cavity or even a large cholesteatoma. They are usually revealed by a rapid development towards suppuration after surgery. Such cholesteatomas can of course be prevented by examining the edges of the perforation and the back of the tympanic cavity under the microscope during consultation and during surgery. Antroscopy may also be considered as a means of avoiding an important mistake. The treatment of cholesteatomas caused by inadequate diagnosis is the same as treatment of other cholesteatomas, as defined in the chapter on indications.

Iatrogenic Cholesteatomas Caused by Faulty Technique

Iatrogenic cholesteatomas are unfortunately a rather common complication of tympanoplasty [41]. In the majority of cases, they take the form of benign pearls which can easily be extracted during a consultation. In about one-third of the cases, they are larger and extend either to the tympanic cavity or to the posterior cavities. In such cases, a second tympanoplasty becomes necessary, possibly using a technique comparable to that used in tympanoplasty for cholesteatoma or epithelialization.

The most important factor favouring the appearance of an iatrognic cholesteatoma is the result of a previous failure. The edge of the epithelium is often far from defined on a graft which is irregularly perforated, partially adherent, displaced in relation to the sulcus and the annulus.

A second factor is the graft in overlay on the lateral surface of the tympanic membrane, i.e. over the de-epithelialized remnant of the tympanic membrane. This, whatever technique is used, involves a risk of leaving a fragment of epithelium under the graft. A convexity of the anterior and inferior wall of the meatus is enough to make it impossible to see a fragment of skin left in the bed of the graft at the angle between the meatus and the tympanic membrane. This is also true if the epithelium is fragile. Complete removal of the anteroinferior skin and the resultant drilling of the bony overhang is not an absolute palliative for such a situation. A graft on the medial surface of the membrane (inlay or underlay) is not a guarantee against an iatrogenic cholesteatoma either, since an error in the dissection of the handle of the malleus may cause the same problems. Nonetheless, inlay grafts placed under the remnants of the tympanic membrane do give rise to fewer iatrogenic cholesteatomas – their disadvantage is rather that they are unstable.

The seat of the iatrogenic cholesteatomas may be the graft, the external auditory meatus or the mastoid, by migration.

Cholesteatomas of the Graft

The most common type of iatrogenic cholesteatoma is juxta-annular or annular. Several varieties may be found. The most benign form is the cholesteatoma caused by insufficiently unrolling the skin placed over the graft, which leads to the formation of a pearl of epithelium lateral to the fascia. The cholesteatoma may also, on the other hand, be medial to the graft, as a result of the inclusion of a fragment of epithelium on the remnants of the tympanic membrane. They are usually situated in the anterior or inferior zone where the angle between the meatus and the tympanic membrane is most difficult to visualize. In such cases it is generally possible to find a medial plane of connective tissue provided by the remaining part of the tympanic membrane (fig. 28, 29).

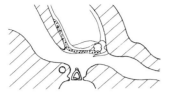 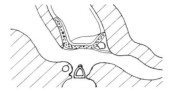

Fig. 28. Iatrogenic cholesteatoma of the graft – superficial cholesteatoma on the annulus caused by insufficiently unrolling the anteroinferior skin. It is generally possible to remove such a cholesteatoma by simple dissection.

Fig. 29. Iatrogenic cholesteatoma of the graft – deeper cholesteatoma on the annulus caused by inadequate deepithelialization of the annulus. Removal by dissection is again generally possible.

A more serious form is the juxta-annular cholesteatoma which breaks into the tympanic cavity into which it extends (fig. 30). This type of cholesteatoma may open, scattering squames which do not become fixed, or it may extend to the tympanic cavity, becoming highly invasive. One of the present authors has encountered an extension beneath the labyrinth and between the facial nerve and the sigmoid sinus in one case, and an anteroinferior extension which had exposed the internal carotid artery in another.

The second variety of cholesteatoma of the graft is the intratympanic cholesteatoma (fig. 31). These may be found on the de-epithelialized remnants of the tympanic membrane in 'overlay' techniques, or on the spatula of the malleus handle in 'overlay' or 'underlay' techniques.

The third variety encountered is the cholesteatoma which has developed in the meatus, under the skin flaps (fig. 32). If the flaps are inadequately unrolled when replaced, this may lead to a flattened cholesteatoma between the skin and the bony canal. The cause may also be a torn flap which rolls up and leads to skin inclusion (fig. 33).

Cholesteatomas Caused by Damage to the
External Auditory Meatus

A cholesteatoma may develop outside the bony external auditory meatus if the meatus was lowered too far during an antro-attico-mastoidectomy, preserving the canal. Another mechanism is osteitis in a

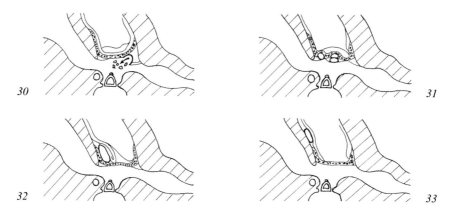

Fig. 30. Iatrogenic cholesteatoma of the graft – cholesteatoma on the annulus which has broken into the tympanic cavity. The whole reconstruction must be done again.

Fig. 31. Iatrogenic cholesteatoma of the graft – intratympanic cholesteatoma. This may occur either on remnants of the tympanic membrane if the graft is placed on the lateral surface, or on the spatula of the malleus handle if the graft is placed on the medial surface.

Fig. 32. Iatrogenic cholesteatoma of the meatus caused by inadequate unrolling of skin flaps.

Fig. 33. Iatrogenic cholesteatoma of the meatus caused by the inclusion of epithelial debris during dissection of the canal skin.

meatus which has been inadequately lined, either with the canal skin or a fascia graft, or, even better, the two together (fig. 34). The skin invaginated into the weak zone and finally forms a large pocket in the mastoid cavity. This can also be caused by a insufficiently hermetic reconstruction of the meatus by cortical bone or cartilage.

Cholesteatomas Caused by 'Transplantation'
This variety is caused by the migration of epithelial debris due to various mechanisms – irrigation, suction, dirty instruments. Their location varies – they may be found in the mastoid cortex, the squamous part of the temporal bone, the soft tissue behind the ear, etc.

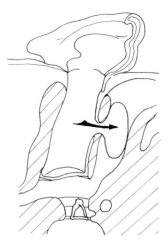

Fig. 34. Iatrogenic cholesteatoma caused by perforation of the bony canal.

Cholesteatomas Following the Insertion of an Aeration Tube

We have observed a cholesteatoma of the tympanic cavity formed by suction of a weak area left by a drain, or by the introduction of epithelial debris. This cholesteatoma, limited to the tympanic cavity and centred around a zone where a transtympanic aeration tube had formerly been inserted, was obviously linked to the tube.

Prevention

In order to prevent iatrogenic cholesteatomas, the surgeon must of course carry out perfect dissections, properly visualized, after controlling the bleeding. He must also preserve the whole of the bony canal. He must avoid premature irrigation and suction in the antrum when the tympanic cavity has not been treated. Finally, when working in areas of mucosa after working in areas of epithelium, he must ensure that his instruments have been perfectly cleaned.

Therapeutic Consequences

Diagnosis of an iatrogenic cholesteatoma must be made as early as possible. A pearl on the anterior or inferior annulus is generally discovered during a follow-up examination in the first or second year after the operation. Simple eradication under the microscope, with or without a local anesthetic, generally ensures a successful removal by enucleation of the pearl and marsupialization of the pocket. This often means an increase in the area of the tympanic membrane which may improve certain types of anterior or inferior obliteration of the angle between the tympanic membrane and the meatus. Hearing may also improve.

If the iatrogenic cholesteatoma is only discovered later, either because there has been no follow-up or because the pearl is located deeper, surgery is usually necessary because the graft has been destroyed and especially because the cholesteatoma has extended into the tympanic cavity. A second type I tympanoplasty is usually sufficient, but it may be necessary to use a closed technique with a posterior tympanotomy or, more rarely, an open technique with obliteration.

Such iatrogenic cholesteatomas may be associated with a graft which is too lateral, and whose medial surface is epithelialized. In this case it is necessary to resect the graft and to use the cholesteatoma matrix lining the meatus laterally to the sulcus and the original annulus as canal skin, or else repeat an anterior obliteration and/or a graft which is too lateral. Iatrogenic cholesteatomas naturally become more difficult to excise if diagnosis is delayed. Even the simplest tympanoplasties and myringoplasties must therefore be followed up every year until the 3rd year, and thereafter every 2 years.

Residual and Recurrent Cholesteatomas

We shall close this chapter on histology with the definitions of two types of cholesteatoma which are the result of unsuccessful tympanoplasty [99, 106, 171, 205, 208, 210, 212, 214, 217, 218], and which we shall be referring to throughout this report. Both are types of recurrent cholesteatoma. A residual cholesteatoma is a recurrence of the tumour, while the retraction pocket is a recurrence of the pathogenesis. International usage draws a clear distinction between the two terms. A residual cholesteatoma is formed from a fragment of matrix, a recurrent cholesteatoma is a retraction pocket.

Residual Cholesteatoma
A residual cholesteatoma is, by definition, a cholesteatoma which has reformed from a fragment of matrix left by the surgeon. Its size depends on two main factors – the size of the residual matrix fragment,

and the time which has elapsed since the operation. The speed of tissue growth may vary depending on age (it is definitely faster in children) and certain inflammatory (mucous otitis) or infectious factors (acute otitis). These residual cholesteatomas generally take the appearance of a pearl. Magnan [132], basing his conclusion on various experimental data, thinks that during the healing process in the middle ear cavities, the connective tissue lining the exposed bony surface surrounds residual epithelial debris. They are caught in the submucous connective tissue and form a microscopic cyst which grows slowly until it becomes visible. This latency implies that a reasonable waiting period before attempting any second-look operation after a tympanoplasty for cholesteatoma would be at least 1 year, and that there should be a routine check of the submucosa whenever the mucosa in thick. The pearl must be removed as a whole with the surrounding mucosa.

Otherwise, the cholesteatoma takes on the much more serious shape of an epidermosis with ill-defined edges, like a spillage of candle. Even despite the excision of the surrounding mucosa, the risk of a recurrence is much greater.

Recurrent Cholesteatoma: the Retraction Pocket

A retraction pocket is a recurrence of the most common process by which cholesteatomas are formed, by a retraction of the canal skin and the tympanic membrane into the bony cavities. It is therefore more especially a complication of closed technique. Tubal insufficiency is definitely the main factor involved in this retraction, but other factors must be taken into account. Sheehy [204] in particular mentions the role of the fibrous tissue linking the new tympanic membrane to the medial wall of the tympanic cavity, especially around the posterior and superior bony annulus. The temporary inclusion of silastic eliminates such adhesions and stabilizes the new tympanic membrane, but does not eliminate all retraction pockets. Most authors stress with Jansen [117] the necessity to reconstruct all notches, whether caused by the lesions or by surgery, with cartilage which has been reshaped or thinned as necessary. However, if the tubal insufficiency becomes more pronounced, the pocket will pass beneath the cartilage reconstruction. Finally, we may also stress the atrophy of fascia, and prefer homografts or perichondrium.

The structure of a retraction pocket may vary. Its usual form is a sac of epithelium lined with connective tissue. It may take the form of a veil of epithelium which is difficult to delimit and to eliminate. A retraction pocket may form sooner or later after the operation. If it is sooner, before the second look, a closed technique tympanoplasty will often be changed into an open technique tympanoplasty with or without obliteration. If it is later, it causes serious problems. It is necessary to judge exactly whether its size is limited or not, and whether it is self-cleansing or not. Some retraction pockets remain stable, their limits easily visible under the microscope. Others become steadily deeper, wearing away the bony canal and can be kept under control. Some pockets, on the other hand, extend rapidly into the depths and form another cholesteatoma, which may be large, within a few years.

Although retraction pockets have been described with closed techniques, they may occur on an open technique, with or without obliteration, but they are less serious in such cases. It is possible, for example, to see a part of the new tympanic membrane extend medially, especially above a reconstructed ossicular chain, to form a pocket extending towards the Eustachian tube. It is obvious that the result is not satisfactory from a functional point of view, but the anatomical risk is to all intents and purposes negligible.

Pathogenesis

The reader may be surprised by such a long chapter on the pathogenesis of cholesteatoma. Many published works on this subject in the last 15 years deserve to be discussed here. They demonstrate not only the desire to investigate precursors of cholesteatoma in order to undertake preventive action, but also the complexity of the various factors which affect such lesions.

We would rather risk beins criticized for repeating ourselves (occasionally) than being too sektchy in our presentation. The following outline has been adopted for this chapter:

General comments
Cholesteatoma: primary or secondary?
The embryonic remnant theory
The epithelial metaplasia hypothesis
The epithelial migration
    The tympanic membrane – a fragile barrier
    Pathogenesis of epithelial migration
    General: papillary growth, cell migration, epithelialization
    The theories: surface migration, deep migration, epithelialization
    and atelectasis, posttraumatic implantation
    Synthesis and role of Eustachian tube malfunction
    Precursors of cholesteatoma

General Comments

Despite its misnomer, cholesteatoma of the middle ear has been a subject of deep interest for a long time, since the mystery of its pathogenesis has not been clarified yet. Certainly, cholesteatoma, like chronic otitis media which may precede, coexist, or occur after it, has various causes. There are so many different parameters involved that it is so difficult to take them all into account at the same time.

First and foremost, cholesteatoma is an anatomico-clinical syndrome which is characterized by the presence of keratinizing, desquamating Malpighian epithelium in the middle ear cavities. If there is no infection, such a presence may be tolerated for a long time – this is the cholesteatoma's 'secret life', which leads, sooner or later, to a situation of conflict. The cholesteatoma's 'public life' becomes apparent either at a comparatively late stage due to the functional impairment caused by its extension, or at an earlier stage due to the infection disturbing the patient.

The simplest definition of cholesteatoma is 'skin in the wrong place' (Gray, 1964). Although it may be criticized as an oversimplification, this aphorism may serve as a practical concept in the study of pathogenesis. It is a general rule that all treatment must be as rational as possible, and be based on pathophysiological data. Unfortunately, in medicine and surgery, treatments complying with this requirement are rare. In this respect, the treatment of cholesteatoma is exemplary.

As Sade [185] stresses, it is difficult to be certain of how each particular cholesteatoma is formed, as few patients are kept under continuous observation. We must all be pragmatical. When 'there is skin in the tympanic cavity', the process is taking place on another level. The lesions are irreversible and must be totally eradicated. This is why, over the last 10 years or so, the idea of the 'precursor of cholesteatoma' has gained popularity, introducing the idea of preventive treatment when faced with certain otoscopic appearances. At present we have no accurate epidemiological statistics to support the idea, but:

(1) Statistics concerning closed chronic seromucous otitis media confirm that there is a cause-and-effect relationship here, but it is not possible to give precise figures. There is no strict parallel between middle ear effusion and the risk of secondary cholesteatoma. Often the intervals between these two aspects last as long as several years, during which the otoscopic examination is almost inevitably interrupted.

(2) Some cholesteatomas, particularly in the attic, develop without suppuration and without any apparent insufficiency of the Eustachian tube. This is attributed to passing or infraclinical inflammatory phenomena in the closed tympanomastoid system.

(3) In all this discussion, there is only one solid, significant fact –

cholesteatoma accounts for 30–40% of cases of chronic otitis media in children, and between 60 and 70% in adults. This can only mean that between 30 and 40% of cases of chronic otitis media in children gradually develop into chronic otitis media with cholesteatoma.

Cholesteatomas – Primary or Secondary?

A lesion is primary when it appears first, before other lesions. For some authors, only the embryonic remnant cholesteatomas of the petrous bone comply with this 'primary' definition (congenital cholesteatoma). From a clinical viewpoint, it is impossible to reject this standard distinction, but we cannot give it a real pathophysiological meaning. There have been many observations of attic cholesteatomas developing without infection, like an epithelial tumour (a true keratoma). Eustachian tube function may be normal, or only becomes affected in the presence of inflammation caused by either the growth or the infection of the cholesteatoma. It is all too easy to blame a prolonged, subclinical insufficiency of the Eustachian tube, which cannot be proved, as a convenient scapegoat. The primary nature of epithelial invasion from the tympanic membrane cannot be denied, even if its progress is facilitated by special anatomical conditions in this area. McGuckin [145] spoke of 'primary nonmalignant destructive ear disease', and Mawson [146] of 'atticoantral disease'. The term 'primary' cannot be applied to retraction pockets which are developing into cholesteatomas, because they are always pathological and themselves secondary. Except in a few special cases, this distinction between primary and secondary cholesteatomas is a conventional clinical description which may acquire a practical usefulness at a later stage in the development of our knowledge. Today, pathogenesis must still be studied under the three classical headings – embryonic remnant, metaplasia and invasion.

Embryonic Remnant Theory

The theory of cholesteatoma as a tumour was put forward by Korner in 1830. Comparing cholesteatomas of the middle ear with intracranial cholesteatomas, he considered them as congenital cysts. The complexity of the formation of the petrous bone and the middle ear in the embryo provided enough theoretical arguments for the inclusion of cells which could become epithelial – the otic vesicle for Mickulicz [cf. 28], the vestibular aqueduct for Bottcher [cf. 28], and the paratympanic organ for Teed [cf. 28]. This was the long favoured theory in France. Later, this was discussed in the English literature. In 1963, Cawthorne [32] argued at length that the frequency of cholesteatomas of congenital origin was underestimated. In 1965, Derlacki and Clemis [56] gave a three-point definition of congenital otomastoid cholesteatoma: (1) development behind and intact tympanic membrane; (2) no history of infection in the ear, an (3) starting-point from inclusions of squamous epithelium or undifferentiated tissue which is transformed into squamous epithelium during the development of the temporal bone.

It must be stated at the outset that such arguments discredit the cause they support by relying on the metaplasia whose mechanism is far from clear. Now that we know more about subclinical retrotympanic effusion, it is not possible to claim seriously that there is no history of infection in the ear. An intact tympanic membrane is significant only relatively. On the contrary, since we know the ease of which the epithelium may migrate unseen, even with just a few cells, we must be absolutely certain that the cholesteatoma is completely independent of the tympanic membrane before we can consider it as congenital. Although the embryonic remnant mechanism cannot be discounted, it is certainly at least as rare as the frequency of the pure intracranial cholesteatoma, in terms of otological extremes. As early as 1925, [149] Nager wrote that primary cholesteatoma of the ear 'is so rare it is of no practical significance for diagnosis and treatment'. Some authors mention the embryonic remnant theory with reference to the branchial origin of the external auditory meatus, out of ignorance of its true development in the embryo. The research of Fleischer [74], and later of Goedbloed [96], has shown that it develops from a solid epithelial plug, which appears subsequently to the disappearance of branchial phenomena. This plug is hollowed by a process of erosion, while a sheet of epithelium, whose ends are long and finger-like, remains in the bottom of the meatus. Hellman as early as 1925 noted that the epithelium is sent out as a long-cell tract as far as under the mucosa of the tympanic cavity, and this was confirmed by Friedman [82]. This appearance persists during development until the dividing line between epithelium and mucosa becomes clearer with the differentiation of the sulcus, the annulus and the collagen layer.

Epithelial Metaplasia Hypothesis

Epithelial metaplasia undoubtedly takes place in the middle ear, both in its mucoid form and its squamous form. The difficulty lies in deciding whether such metaplasia can give rise to a cholesteatoma. In 1873, Wendt [cf. 28] thought it could. Since 1976, Sade and Halevy [191] have developed many arguments to bring this theory up to date. We are indebted to them for much of this section. The most recent data provided by cell biology have made ideas of cell specificity less rigid. We know that the chromosome equipment of every cell still contains potentially all the original genetic information, but during development, the information in each cell becomes more precise and more specific, and then deteriorates. Each cell is programmed to synthesize a given protein by the activation of a section of its stock of DNA (operon), while the operons which are coded for other proteins are blocked. Although anything seems possible, in particular in vitro, cell differentiation in vivo is still a restricting process, especially for tissue with highly specialized functions, such as nerve tissue or liver. Epithelial cells are less well protected and, like haematopoietic cells, receive a large amount of information from the external environment which may influence their functioning and therefore their morphology. Their rate of renewal varies and dead cells are eliminated by disposal into body cavities, the mucociliary system or desquamation; the renewal thus comes from 'stem' cells. Lymphoid cells, for example, become morphologically and functionally differentiated in several directions as a result of many factors – embryonic induction, information received from organs through which they have passed, pathological stimulation, etc. The same is true, in vivo, for the basal cells of the epithelium. They cannot code the synthesis of protein which is too far from the direction which they have taken in differentiation. They do however retain a relative freedom – to differentiate into any of the different types of epithelial-covering cells. In normal conditions, maturation after mitosis occurs in perfect harmony. There is a well-balanced proportion of, for example, 1 mucus cell to 5 or 10 ciliated cells. In a sheep's stomach, we can find granules of mucus and keratohyalin together in the same cell. In humans, vaginal epithelium synthesizes keratohyalin during the follicular phase and mucus during the luteal phase of the menstrual cycle. In the larynx and the oesophagus, stratified squamous epithelium progresses with age. In pathological conditions mucus cells may become predominant. In other cases, flattened, epidermoid-type cells, which become capable of synthesizing keratin, may appear. A number of experiments (Walbach, Melanby and Fell, McLaughlin, Sweeny) have been reported by Sade [186], all showing the influence of different factors favouring epidermoid epithelial metaplasia: (a) lack of vitamin A; (b) addition of oestrogens to the environment; (c) influence of the mesenchyme associated with the epithelium in animals, gizzard mesenchyme favours mucous metaplasia, while hypodermic mesenchyme favours keratinization; (d) an increase in CO^2 content favours mucous metaplasia.

In the Ear

It thus seems that the genetic information contained in basal cells can be modified by information from the surrounding environment (changes in O_2 and CO_2 contents) as well as by metabolic phenomena coded in the connective tissue. Synthesis of mucus and of keratin nonetheless seem to be mutually exclusive, and it is difficult to explain the presence of stratified squamous epithelium juxtaposed to mucous cells in the same biopsy. If a higher CO_2 content seems to be an important factor in mucous metaplasia, does this not argue against the metaplastic theory of cholesteatoma? We think that the basic data at present at our disposal allow two answers:

Epidermoid metaplasia is not rare in chronic otitis media. For Sade [185] it is present in 60% of cases.

Before the introduction of cell cultures, authors had considered the metaplastic hypothesis for the origin of cholesteatoma, and this was confirmed by the continuing use of ambiguous nomenclature – cholesteatosis (black or white), cholesterin granuloma, epidermic or epidermoid metaplasia.

Bremond et al. [26] express the problem clearly: 'Metaplasia of the lining of the middle ear is always epidermoid and not epithelial.' Friedman [82] speaks of 'nonkeratinizing squamous epithelium', and Sade [186] of 'simple stratified squamous epithelium'. It is in fact stratified pavement epithelium, but having no stratum granulosum or stratum corneum. There is usually a gradual transition from normal mucosa. It is difficult to base any argument, as Sade does, on a few rare histological sections which show a sudden change in type of epithelium – sections are two-dimensional, and misleading impressions may be given, depending on the plane of the section. It is true that, in this epidermoid metaplasia, keratin-synthesizing cells may appear [22, 186], but they are rare and sparsely distributed. Epidermoid metaplasia of the middle ear does not seem likely to give rise to the formation of a cholesteatoma. It is impossible to apply results obtained experimentally in animals to humans, given that spontaneous cholesteatomas occur very rarely in animals, and that it is extremely difficult to induce cholesteatomas experimentally (all experimental cholesteatomas are in fact caused by migration). The essential argument is based on conventional histology and electronic microscopy. Cholesteatoma is formed by an epithelial, not an epidermoid, lining. This epithelium includes all types of keratinocytes linked by desmosomes, as well as Langerhans' and Merkel's cells which prove that it is indeed skin. Moreover, Lim et al. [125] have observed melanocytes in the matrix. We refer the reader to the article by Sade [185] for arguments that cholesteatomas of the medial attic are cysts of metaplastic origin which open secondarily into the meatus. It is difficult to imagine how metaplastic mucosa can be homogeneous enough to form a cleavable epithelial cyst, especially when the attic happens to be the area where metaplastic phenomena are the least common. How is it possible to explain, when the pathogenic phenomena are exactly similar, that there are no cholesteatomas of the paranasal sinuses, apart from a few dubious examples mentioned in the literature on the subject? It is, of course, always possible to attribute this to the inductive influence of the accompanying mesenchyme, which is different. This shows that the metaplastic theory is based on dialectical and specious arguments which cannot, theoretically, be totally rejected. It does however raise an important problem – the justification of closed techniques and even open-techniques tympanoplasty with 'management' of the tympanic cavity. In the present state of our operative observations, we do not think that this can affect our ideas of the surgical treatment of cholesteatoma today.

The Epithelial Migration

Standard theory classifies epithelial migration according to the way in which it takes place:

(1) Direct invasion: from the edges of a perforation (invasion theory upheld by Habermann [cf. 28] as early as 1928. Schuknecht [197]

has shown, on routine temporal bone sections, that the epithelium crosses the edges of tympanic perforations much more commonly than is generally admitted. This situation may show no clinical sign.

Palva [155] has demonstrated this type of invasion in 11 out of 13 temporal bones of which serial sections were examined, but without the formation of a cholesteatoma although the epithelium may extend over a considerable distance into the middle ear. The dividing line between the epithelium and the mucosa is generally clear cut, but there may exist in places a transitional type of epithelium which could suggest metaplasia. In a few cases, there is a clear dividing line between the two epithelia, but the squamous epithelium may send out finger-like extensions which undermine the chorion of the neighbouring mucosa and form parakeratotic pearls. A cholesteatoma begins to form as soon as the keratin debris is no longer evacuated towards the meatus or the Eustachian tube.

(2) Invagination was mentioned by Wittmack whose name is still linked with the pathogenesis of cholesteatoma. In our opinion the mechanism of retraction pockets is the same in the pars flaccida as in the pars tensa.

(3) Papillary growth of the basal layer of the epithelium was demonstrated by Ruedi [cf. 28] and Friedman [82], especially in experimental cholesteatomas. Acanthosis with the formation of parakeratotic pearls is now a familiar process.

(4) Cell implantation is another possibility, as is shown by cholesteatomas occurring after fractures of the petrous bone. There is incontrovertible evidence that paracentesis or the insertion of transtympanic aeration tubes may be to blame – the tympanic membrane may heal behind cells imprisoned in this way. This cell implantation may even occur spontaneously in the pars tensa when inflammation and/or infection locally destroys the mucosa on the medial surface of the tympanic membrane and the layer of collagen. A few cells from the basal layer of the epithelium may migrate, helped by the inflammatory reaction. We know how far the mucosa of the medial surface of the tympanic membrane may be modified in cases of secretory chronic otitis media. Iatrogenic cholesteatomas are now familiar, and unfortunately too much so, having a quasi-experimental value being due to an error of technique in general. But, in a considerable number of cases, it may be thought that a pre-existing subclinical invasion may not have been recognized.

We have listed these hypotheses in order not to depart from standard theory, but no single one of them can explain all the cases. When patients seek medical advice, most of them already have a fully constituted cholesteatoma. It is true that since microscopic examination of the tympanic membrane in routine check-ups has become widespread, otologists have been able to increase observations of patients who have been regularly followed up, and in whom they have seen cholesteatomas form over the years.

We are no longer in the realm of theory, but in the realm of incontrovertible clinical facts, when we speak of the idea of a precursor of cholesteatoma. If we wish to improve the treatment we can offer, we must be able to reconstruct the pathophysiological process. Why does the squamous epithelium of the external auditory meatus occupy the tympanomastoid cavities? Does it have a particular dynamism? Is it invasive? Or is it attracted? Why does cholesteatoma occur in some patients, while the others, with exactly the same clinical and otoscopic conditions, only have simple chronic otitis media or apparently stable scar sequelae? Why does it so often occur in both ears?

Tympanic Membrane – A Fragile Barrier

The tympanic membrane is a delicate barrier which is easily destabilized. There is no other part of the body comparable to the tympanic membrane, which is composed of an extremely thin sheet of connective tissue with a different lining on each surface – epithelial on the lateral surface, mucous on the medial. Its mechanical resistance is low, it is poorly vascularized and, in normal conditions, its metabolic activity is slight. In a pathological context it offers little resistance to the progress of inflammation or infection and the characteristics of the cavities which it encloses favour chronic disease. These attacks only have to be intense and/or prolonged, and the lesions will soon become irreversible. Above all, the otologist must always bear in mind that the tympanic membrane is the seat of a generally centrifugal migration of cells from the malleus handle as has been shown in the research carried out by Litton [129, 130] and Alberti [8]. This migration carries on in the same direction, which explains the piling up of cell debris in the fundi of retraction pockets and operative cavities if their shape does not allow proper self-cleansing. We shall go on to examine a few detailed points concerning this barrier, in which two different types of tissue are placed back-to-back, almost in a situation of conflict.

In the Pars flaccida

The connective tissue separating the two epithelia is areolar and almost nonexistent in 50% of cases. The squamous epithelium is often depressed around the notch of Rivinus. Schwartz [199] has shown that some depressions of the pars flaccida, with transitional forms leading to cholesteatoma, are often bilateral and hereditary. Marquet [138] and one of the present authors, on the other hand, have stressed that some patients have a fairly well organized fibrillated connective layer in the pars flaccida, as can be observed during tympanotomies for otosclerosis or the removal of homografts. Individuals with this kind of anatomical particularity undoubtedly run less risk of having a cholesteatoma.

The previous authors raised the possibility that there could be perforations of the pars flaccida and sometimes mentioned chronic atticitis in the absence of cholesteatoma [131]. In reality, this is a purely artificial distinction. Any perforation of the pars flaccida is edged, histologically, by squamous epithelium from the meatus. In some cases, total epithelialization of Prussak's pouch may be completely concealed by a keratinized squame from the tympanic membrane. It must be considered that 'attic lesions = cholesteatoma'.

Resistance of the Pars tensa Is Not Uniform

The posterosuperior subligamentary region is particularly thin and fragile. This is where the vast majority of marginal perforations and retraction pockets are to be found. In many cases such retraction pockets form a cap over the head of the stapes after eroding the long process of the incus. Even if there is no infection, the wall of the pocket may disappear in places – we then find a posterosuperior perforation with a 'tongue' of epithelium forming a bridge between the malleus or the tympanomalleolar ligament and the head of the stapes. Sometimes the epithelium covering the superstructure of the stapes may even have lost all contact with its starting-point. An observer may speak of invasive epidermosis although the initial condition was in fact a limited pocket of atelectasis which subsequently broke. Such developments must have been observed by every attentive otologist, especially if he has taken the trouble to make detailed sketches of the otoscopic appearance.

This localized fragility varies from case to case, depending on the quality of the connective layer of the tympanic membrane. Individual anatomical peculiarities may accentuate this fragility. The fibrocartilaginous annulus of the tympanic membrane does not have the same dimensions around the whole circumference of the membrane. It becomes thinner superiorly and posteriorly and disappears gradually towards the posterior spur of the tympanic bone. This petering out occurs at varying distances from the posterior insertion of the tympanic-malleolar ligament, and sometimes even at this insertion. There may be an actual hiatus between the two. Given the importance of the annular fibrocartilage in inducing the formation of the collagen fibres in the tympanic membrane, it is obvious that this is an area of weakness, where there will be no spontaneous healing if there is a perforation, where retraction is easier, and where the epithelium may enter supported by the chorda tympani.

Along the annulus, especially in its inferior portion, the anteroinferior part of the tympanic membrane is the last area to adhere. Retraction pockets or pockets of complete atelectasis generally start in the posterosuperior quadrant and extend to the paracentral, and then the premalleolar regions. The tympanic epithelium, which has been 'orphaned' by the loss of its supporting collagen, lines the tympanic cavity as if seeking a new support, and will do so all the more easily if there is a residual negative pressure. It may line the hypotympanum and even the orifice of the Eustachian tube, while a crescent-shaped portion remains for a long time in the normal plane of the membrane.

At this stage, the epithelium lining the tympanic cavity may become detached and give rise to what appears to be a sharp-edged perforation through which a disc of epithelium can be seen on the promontory. In a retraction pocket, or in more complete atelectasis, the epithelium will coil up in the tympanic cavity and mould itself more or less to the walls. It remains capable of being detached easily over a long period, as can be shown by tubal insufflation, then starts to adhere to certain areas, generally in the following order: incudostapedial region, promontory, posterior part of the mesotympanum, medial surface of the remains of the collagen layer of the tympanic membrane. As long as there is no accumulation of epithelial debris, we cannot speak of a cholesteatoma, but there are many fine distinctions, and the intermediate stages are difficult to judge, even for an experienced otologist.

In the middle ear, the epithelium may behave differently, depending on circumstances which vary from patient to patient, due to: (a) individual anatomical variations, especially in the mucous folds and ligaments; (b) Eustachian tube function; (c) inflammatory reactions which vary from one individual to another and depend on the bacteria involved in the superinfection, the age and hygiene of the patient and the quality of the mesenchyma, and (d) behaviour of the mucosa.

It is rare to find the mucosa coming to meet the epithelium. This may be the case when a hyperplastic promontory comes into contact with the edges of a paracentral kidney-shaped perforation. In this case, the epithelium will be on the same level. When there is extensive atelectasis, the phenomenon which seems to be the most important in the development of the cholesteatoma is the accumulation of epithelial debris when the retraction pocket or the atelectasis loses its self-cleansing capacity. This is the 'turning-point' in the life of the ear. Quite apart from whatever may determine the speed with which surface epithelial cells are renewed, it appears that the development of a cholesteatoma is linked to the accumulation of cell debris and the loss of the self-cleansing capacity. This accumulation may be aggravated by inflammation when it comes into contact with the basal layer. In fact, the most important factor, allowing the accumulation of desquamated cell debris, is the aeration coefficient of the retraction pocket – the ratio between its volume and the area open at its neck. We know very little about most of the factors which control cell migration, but the research of Sakai et al. [193] is very interesting: with the aim of checking the comparative behaviour of the epithelium of the meatus and that of the cholesteatoma matrix, they studied various fragments in a culture. It appeared that epithelium of the meatus migrated at a rate of between 7 and 10 mm in 10 days, while cells of the matrix only covered between 0 and 3 mm over the same period. But in both cases the migration is centrifugal and remains so in the culture. It is therefore easy to understand that lesions of the attic are particularly favourable to the development of a cholesteatoma. The ossicles serve initially as a support for the epithelium, whether from a retraction pocket, a flap in need of a support, or an epidermosis. Their almost nonexistent periosteum and the paucity of their blood supply mean that they cannot hold out indefinitely – which explains the fact that the short process of the incus or the superstructure of the stapes are more commonly eroded. The mucosal folds and ligaments, the chorda tympani and any granulomata which may be present, are ideal starting-points for this 'wandering' "epithelium" in search of a mate'. Anything may happen in such cases and, unlike Sade [186], we are not surprised to see the medial attic lined first. In the external auditory meatus, certain conditions favour the destabilization of the epithelium – heat, moisture, a lack of aeration and potential infection. These conditions are well known to dermatologists. The otologist can judge accurately the influence of the narrowness of the meatus or the hyperplasia of the temporal bone on postoperative results. Some even suggest a routine widening of the meatus [77].

Pathogenesis of Epithelial Migration

It is no longer possible to consider epithelial migration as a theory, i.e. an abstract idea, or an intellectual hypothesis. It is a clinical and experimental fact. From a clinical viewpoint, the regular microscopic examinations of certain patients have shown beyond any doubt that the initially self-cleansing retraction pockets can become typical cholesteatomas. One of the present authors has observed the gradual formation of a cholesteatoma in the attic 8 years after the closure of a paracentral perforation under the influence of negative pressure persisting in the tympanic cavity, and without the possibility of attributing the cholesteatoma to an iatrogenic factor.

Experimentally, in 1959, Ruedi [182] showed that an irritant, applied to the medial surface of the tympanic membrane, favoured epithelial invasion of the tympanic cavity in guinea pigs. In 1969, Fernandez and Lindsay [70] confirmed this demonstration and showed that a lesion of the fibrous layer of the tympanic membrane or the chorion of the pars flaccida was enough to make the epithelial invasion possible. The fact that the tympanic membrane is intact does not thus constitute an argument against the epithelial migration hypothesis. Recently, using various procedures and various irritants with rabbits, Steinbach [227] confirmed the possibility that experimental cholesteatomas developed preferentially in the posterosuperior region. He stressed that disturbance of the ventilation in the meatus or the tympanic cavity, which are important in humans, is not essential in animals. All the research therefore points to the importance of a direct lesion of the collagen layer of the medial surface of the tympanic membrane by an irritant (talcum, histoacryl or salicylic acid). For a long time, cholesteatoma was thought to be peculiar to man. Chole et al. [43] have recently published a report on the Mongolian gerbil *(Meriones unguiculatis)* which develops spontaneous cholesteatoma with bony erosion in 45% of ears of animals aged between 1 and 2 years.

General Comments

Despite this incontrovertible evidence, when a patient first seeks medical advice, the lesions are already well developed (the 'secret life' and the 'public life' of the cholesteatoma). This has led some authors (fewer and fewer nowadays) to dispute the mechanism which produces a perforation and whether a cholesteatoma is primary or secondary. The fact that closed-tympanic cholesteatomas were seen with little or no defence reaction from the structures of the middle ear has long created a powerful argument in favour of the dysembryoplastic origin of cholesteatoma. We have seen many otologists make false comparisons with the branchial apparatus; although, in fact, the epithelium of the tympanic and pretympanic membrane is governed by a particular embryonic induction, its intensity, being chronobiologically controlled, decreases with age. The epithelium, which comes into contact with the mucosa of the middle ear, has the strategic advantage of this dynamism linked to a particular type of genetic induction. When one considers (in depth) the existence of closed tympanic cholesteatomas, which may be surprising at first, it can easily be explained in the light of these ideas, and depends on two facts, namely (1) there can be no epithelial growth without a connective substratum, and (2) the metabolism of the tympanic membrane is normally slow and not intense. We all know of cases in which spontaneous atrophy of the tympanic membrane has led to extensive loss of substance: this is difficult to explain, as they sometimes heal contrary to expectations.

Inflammation involving the chorion of the mucosa of the tympanic cavity or collagen layer of the tympanic membrane, may activate its epithelium: this has been observed in activated retraction pockets. This mechanism has led some authors to suggest that irritating the edges of small perforations could favour healing. Normally the collagen layer of the tympanic membrane holds it in shape 'like the ribs of an umbrella', the area between are practically acellular. As soon as inflammation occurs, the histological picture changes dramatically, as the organization of the fibres is disturbed, or even destroyed, while the inflammatory cells with the usual macrophages appear.

It has been shown in practice that, during this phase, three invasion mechanisms may occur – papillary growth, disordered cell migration (or epidermosis), and epithelialization by collapse (which we shall the organization of the fibres is disturbed, or even destroyed, while the consider in due course). When the tympanic membrane is open, and, in the absence of any infection or inflammation, the epithelium and the mucosa may remain in position indefinitely, i.e., there is a 'nonaggression pact'. Sometimes it takes several years before a tongue of epithelium can be seen progressing from the posterior tympanomalleolar ligament towards the incudostapedial region. It is also common to find the epithelium going round the malleus handle, although this is difficult to see without careful microscopic examination. It is characteristic, though uncommon, to find a column of epithelium 'like a pile of dishes' forming from the umbo of the malleus. Sometimes, routine examination of the medial surface of the tympanic membrane during simple myringoplasty may revel a large area of pearly epithelium, starting from the edges of the perforation and often covering a tympanosclerotic plaque. Operative techniques should take this into account.

When the mucosa of the tympanic cavity is infected or inflamed, granulomata and polyps precede the epithelium, serving as a bridgehead for the invasion of the tympanic cavity. Histopathological microscopic examination shows this: the specimen may contain mucosa, which may be more or less metaplastic, together with the characteristic epithelium (side-by-side). We stress these aspects, which are familiar to so many otologists, because they may be interpreted in different ways. Those, who uphold the metaplastic theory, emphasize that (1) islands of keratin-synthesizing stratified squamous epithelium may be found well away from the tympanic membrane, therefore making it possible to mistake the epithelial nature for epidermoid metaplasia, and (2) epithelial migration is not an aggressive process which destroys other cells to take their place. Mixed tissue cultures, in which respiratory mucosa is placed in contact with the epithelium, show that a clearcut dividing-line forms between the two, probably by contact inhibition. In fact, there is no question of the epithelium destroying the mucosa directly as K lymphocytes can do to some cells. There is rather a replacement of the mucosa which disappears in front of the epithelium, and does so all the more easily when the mucosa is thinner and less differentiated. This is the case for the mucosa of the attic and the antrum, while the mucosa of the promontory holds out longer. In vitro, there may be contact inhibition at the edge between the two types of epithelium. But we must not be too hasty in assuming that the same will happen in vivo. In the ear, the two are normally in contact, and the squamous epithelium is the seat of inductive dynamism which is characteristic in the normal histological picture. It may slide between the bone and the mucosa. When the epithelium and the mucosa are edge-to-edge, there is bound to be a conflict between the two. This edge cannot be compared either to the maintenance of the status quo found in vitro, or to the genetically controlled limits of natural orifices (the mucous edge of the lip, for example).

In an excellent article, Jackson and Lim [109] report on their research into the ultrastructural morphology of the junction between epithelium and mucosa in human cholesteatomas, and in experimental cholesteatomas in cats. The inflammation which is so common at the dividing line between the two epithelia is favoured by the absence of any really solid connective tissue at this point. At the edge of the advancing squamous epithelium, the migrating epithelial cells are the deepest lying spiny cells and not the basal cells. The migrating cells develop hemidesmosomes which make contact with the basement membrane, and fibrin, which acts as a guide. They are immediately followed by the epithelium which is thickened at this point – the stratum spinosum comprises 12 cells with many mitoses (instead of the normal 5 cells).

A certain balance may be established between two types of epithelium in vivo as well as in vitro, especially if they are normally fairly close to each other. Clinically and experimentally, the aggressive behaviour of the cholesteatoma depends more on infectious and inflammatory phenomena than on the inherent characteristics of the cholesteatomatous epithelium itself, although the possibility immune-type tissue reactions cannot be excluded. The involvement of the connective tissue, however, appears to be essential – skin implanted into a cat's bulla does not form an epithelial pearl, but a morula-type formation which disappears under the influence of a pseudoglandular reaction of the mucosa.

It may be useful to mention here an interesting phenomenon which bas been observed by a number of authors [219] – the possibility that a small island of epithelium, which has purposely been left in place, during a closed-technique operation, on a fistula of the lateral semicircular canal or the oval window for example, may disappear. A year later, during the second look, a very thorough histological examination may show that all traces of any epidermoid element have disappeared. Phagocytosis? Cell erosion? The epithelium was probably composed of elements which were incapable of further multiplication (keratinocytes which had evolved too far). It is a rare occurrence, and although it may be important from a theoretical point of view, this must not be allowed to serve as an excuse for residual cholesteatomas, especially in the posterior tympanic cavity. In some paracentral perforations, especially accompanied by tympanosclerosis, the mucous epithelium curls round the edges of the perforation into the meatus [197]. The problem is thus one of the relationship between the epithelium and the underlying structures on which it rests – in normal conditions (collagen fibres, more or less organized connective tissue, or the fibrocartilage of the annulus) and in pathological conditions (ossicles, mucous folds and ligament mucosa of the tympanic cavity or bone).

Why does this dividing-line become destabilized? Does the epithelial matrix possess special properties? Is inflammation essential? Do changes of pressure in the tympanic cavity predominate? It is clear that all these mechanisms play a synergic role in the typical forms of the fully-formed sac cholesteatoma. But some factors must predominate during the initial period, which varies from one clinical form to another. Retraction pockets probably follow different rules of development from those followed by closed-tympanic cholesteatomas, or by invasive epidermosis. As we have already stated, cholesteatoma is an anatomico-clinical syndrome characterized by the presence of keratinizing and desquamating Malpighian epithelium in the middle ear cavities.

Theories Which Have Been Put Forward

Surface Migration
In 1870, Burnett [cf. 28] noticed that the epithelium of the external auditory meatus had the ability to migrate laterally. In 1890, Habermann and Bezold envisaged the possibility that cholesteatoma might be formed in this way. Politzer noted that the cholesteatoma matrix was continuous with the epithelium of the meatus, especially in the posterosuperior area of the annulus, where the skin of the meatus was

thicker and most vascularized. At this site the vessels are perpendicular to the edge of the bony annulus, thus guiding the migration [127]. Alberti's [8] research confirmed the concept of this centrifugal migration of epithelium from the tympanic membrane and the pretympanic membrane, which tend to become reversed when there is a perforation, in accordance with the general rules of skin healing. The speed of this migration is approximately 50 times faster than the speed of desquamation is in the form of complete horny layers which are cleavable tangentially from the stratum spinosum. When the fibrous layer of the tympanic membrane is still present, this advance is slow and laborious. The junction between epithelium and the mucosa is still most commonly situated around the edges of a central perforation. On the other hand, Schuknecht [197] considers that, in cases with marginal perforation, this line may become established between 1 and 4 mm inside the middle ear.

Starting from the handle of the malleus or from the posterior tympanomalleolar ligament, a flap of epithelium may be supported by the short process of the incus. Sometimes, especially when inflammation is present, the tympanic cavity is invaded by dispersed cells which join up subsequently (epidermosis).

Deep Migration

Ruedi [181] has shown that the cells from the basal layer of the skin could migrate into the underlying connective tissue, with hyperacanthosis, and the formation of epithelial cones and horny globes which proliferate on their own. This is what Schwartz suggests as the form of papillary cholesteatoma. The mechanism is much rarer in the pars tensa, where the squamous epithelium somehow retains the ability to form little balls of epithelium, which were observed by Politzer: this formation may be favoured by certain surgical operations, e.g. tympanoplasty. There may still be a disorderly migration of cells to the medial surface of the pars tensa following a limited modification of its collagen layer, caused by the formation of a granuloma of the mucosa of the tympanic cavity for example.

Epithelialization and Atelectasis

The accumulation of clinical and otoscopic data on ears that have been followed up over a long period has made it possible to describe a progressive condition – the atelectatic tympanic membrane – which may lead to the epithelialization of the tympanic cavity. The terminology, which has been used, varies greatly – collapse of the tympanic membrane, retraction pocket, tympanic retraction, adhesive otitis and even pulsion diverticulum (!). These different names show that there is no unanimous agreement on the pathogenic mechanism, which is, however, even more complex than the terminology would lead us to suppose. We shall adopt the convention of using the term of atelectatic ear whenever the tympanic membrane is atrophic and either wholly or partly situated medially to its normal position. This includes any of the intermediate stages from the most typical posterosuperior retraction pocket to the total collapse of the squamous epithelium. The tympanic membrane is atrophic and the collagen fibres have disappeared as if they had been 'erased'. Their disappearance is not merely theoretical because it has been observed after recurrent seromucous otitis media. This is what Bremond [25] calls the 'disarmed tympanic membrane'. As far as possible, we shall avoid using the term 'adhesive otitis', as this might prejudge the state of the tissue surrounding the residual lumen of the tympanic cavity. In the pure form of atrophic retraction pocket, insufflation or Valsalva manoeuvres will temporarily reverse the collapse. The fixation of squamous epithelium on the incudostapedial region or the promontory is secondary. The situation is not the same when the mucosa of the tympanic cavity undergoes a hyperplastic, later fibrous, inflammatory transformation: it would seem reasonable to suppose that these changes are responsible for actively retracting the tympanic membrane. Any of the intermediate stages is also possible. A cholesteatoma of the attic can sometimes be seen alongside a tympanic cavity filled with fibrosis.

In general, we shall use the term 'atelectasis' without wishing to prejudice the composition of the gaseous contents of the middle ear, since the reduction in the volume of the tympanic cavity is obvious, and, this condition is certainly due to Eustachian tube insufficiency in the widest sense of the term. In reality, it is difficult to assess the share of responsibility that the inflammatory phenomena and the inadequate 'middle ear' aeration hold, since they are closely connected, and one may follow the other. We shall not remind the reader of the complex pathogenic problems posed by retrotympanic seromucous effusions, within intact tympanic membrane. These are the same as for atelectatic ears, but occur at different stages of development. The average age of sufferers with seromucous otitis media is 10 years, whereas the average age of patients with atelectic ears is 27 years, similar to patients with simple chronic suppurative otitis media or cholesteatoma [186]. During the course of seromucous otitis media, the opposite ear is normal in only 20% of cases, the rest being affected by atelectasis in 62%, by a central perforation in 13%, and by attic cholesteatoma in 4%.

During the course of the cholesteatoma, one of the present authors has observed diseases in the opposite ears: 14% cholesteatomas, 9% simple chronic suppuration otitis media, 6% retraction pockets and 3% progressive seromucous otitis. During the development of the cholesteatoma, inflammatory phenomena seem to predominate, and are associated with both the severity and the duration of the Eustachian tube insufficiency. When an aeration tube is inserted, normal conditions are restored. A central perforation with aeration may have a role in stabilizing the ear. The reaction of tissues of an individual to the inflammation is an essential factor in the development of cholesteatoma and it would be inaccurate to say that mechanical factors can explain everything. We may cite as proof the fact that those with facial clefts in childhood suffer almost constantly from tubotympanic problems, which often become stabilized in adulthood, with sequelae of varying degrees of importance. Yet the percentage of cholesteatomas is very moderate. Thus it may be said that 'it is not given to everybody to have a cholesteatoma', even if he suffers from a dysfunction of the Eustachian tube. When atelectasis is constitued, just before puberty, middle ear pressure probably takes over the leading role. As Sade [186] stresses, the inflammatory phenomena have led to the atrophy of the collagen framework of the tympanic membrane, leaving it vulnerable to any negative pressure. Later still, although Eustachian tube function may have improved to a certain extent, other problems appear. These are linked to the repercussions of the atelectasis on the self-cleansing mechanism of the squamous epithelium of the external auditory meatus and will depend: (a) on the extent of the tympanic retraction; (b) on its location, and (c) on any superinfection, which is more likely to be from the outside of this stage.

The mechanical force provided by the migration of cells from the malleus handle is very small, and the slightest surface irregularity is an obstacle to the cleansing of epithelial debris. The existence of small horns of epithelium on the short process of the malleus is a good example of this. The accumulation of debris depends on the narrowness of the neck of the retraction pocket in relation to its volume. Accumulation is definitely favoured in the pars flaccida. The bony annulus superoposteriorly, and the fibrous annulus inferiorly often form an overhang in relation to the fundus of the retraction pocket. The accumulation of epithelial debris favours inflammatory reactions and thus the appearance of granulomata, which may exacerbate the vicious circle – desquamation, accumulation, superinfection, and so on.

Implantation of Epithelium

Implantation is valuable in showing how cholesteatoma originates. There have been rare cases in which cholesteatomas have been observed after fractures of the petrous bone, owing undoubtedly to a pinching of the epithelium of the external auditory meatus in the line of the fracture [64, 86, 254]. Iatrogenic cholesteatomas [41, 127], after myringoplasty or the insertion of an aeration tube [29, 93, 198], are now well known. We have seen several cases of spontaneous grafts of squamous epithelium on to the promontory from a 'pile of dishes' formation starting from the umbo of the tympanic membrane. Even cholesteatoma induced by a stapedectomy is possible [66].

Synthesis

We do not think that the metaplastic theory or the congenital theory can influence our ideas of treatment of a cholesteatoma of the middle ear. The former is not backed up by proof – it is hardly even a hypothesis. The latter concerns a few rare cases, and in no way modifies the therapeutic approach. Is it necessary to use the word 'theory' in connection with the migration of squamous epithelium from the meatus? It is rather an incontrovertible fact. Let us rather concentrate on some explanations. We are still not able to predict or differentiate, given the same anatomico-clinical conditions, which patient will develop cholesteatoma and which will develop tympanosclerosis or adhesive otitis [28]. The authors of the Report to the French ENT Congress in 1966 drew up a vast synoptic table showing the causes of the various forms of progressive or sequelary chronic otitis media. Apart from a few modifications, this table is widely accepted. The destabilization of the tympanic membrane depends on a combination of four factors which are difficult to analyse for every case:

Reactivity of the Lateral Tympanic Epithelium

This is a very special type of epithelium, which is influenced by: (a) genetic induction factors, which affect the type and rate of the centrifugal migration; (b) its relations with the activity of the basal layer; (c) the behaviour of the underlying mesenchyme which, apart from its own activity, transmits information from the mucosa of the tympanic cavity; (d) infection from outside favoured by maceration, and linked to the quality of the cerumen and size of the meatus.

It is possible that a thorough biochemical research on the epithelium of the matrix might provide us with new ideas about normal physiological keratinization in this area. Broekaert et al. stress that cholesteatoma is characterized by the breaking down of the stratum corneum, whereas the main stages in the synthesis of keratin are roughly comparable to those of the skin.

Reactivity of the Mucosa of the Tympanic Cavity and the Mastoid

It is all too easy to blame everything on a nonpatent Eustachian tube and the consequences of this on middle ear pressure. With identical values, and the same duration, no two ears will react alike [136]. On the degree of modification of the mucosa, this will depend, among other things, on the composition of the gaseous contents of the middle ear and gas exchange in the mucosa, thus having an indirect effect on tubal patency. The patency of the Eustachian tube, although initially adequate, may subsequently be influenced by the extent to which the mucosa reacts, and this in turn will depend on the nature of the bacteria or virus, and its epidemic character. Finally, there are, in children, particular conditions which bring together:

(a) *Immunological factors:* the immune system is set up gradually, starting in the first few months of life. In the early stages, it must be integrate outside attacks, but it only reaches complete maturity as puberty approaches, and the importance of hormone regulation of inflammatory reactions is well known;

(b) *Physiological factors:* the composition of the gas in the tympanic cavity, the quality of the mucous secretions, the efficiency of the mucociliary lining are all fundamentally important, but are not always taken sufficiently into account by otologists before they make a decision on treatment. The same is true of the nasal passages, which must be fully patent, not only anatomically, but also functionally; and,

(c) *Anatomical factors:* the position of the Eustachian tube, its narrowness, the possible inadequacy of the velopharyngotubal muscle band are important points which deserve special mention. Cholesteatoma in children is doubtless no different from cholesteatoma in adults from a histological point of view, and many authors are of the opinion that it should receive the same surgical treatment as for adults. It would however be a grave mistake to act in this way in all cases, and to draw no practical conclusions from the above, especially since factors linked to the reactivity of the mucosa and the connective tissue are just as important in children, for quite a long time at least, as dysfunction of the Eustachian tube.

Eustachian Tube Dysfunction

Eustachian tube dysfunction plays an essential role in the pathophysiology of the ear. If it is taken merely as a synonym for obstruction, this will make a proper understanding of the problem impossible. Two important points must be made: (a) severe obstruction, occurring quickly, triggers off considerable reactions in the mucosa. Barotrauma is a typical example. In ordinary seasonal diseases, active inflammatory phenomena predominate over purely functional phenomena, and (b) different authors assess the importance of Eustachian tube function during the course of a cholesteatoma in different ways. In most cases it is difficult to examine because of anatomical changes. Patency of the Eustachian tube is generally not seriously affected and does allow just enough exchange of gases to avoid the appearance of telltale clinical signs. Being of long duration, it still favours sufficient inflammatory activity to cause a slow and inconspicuous atrophy of the collagen layer of the tympanic membrane. An increase in the compliance of the weakened membrane may govern subsequent developments. Flisberg (cf 28) has shown that negative pressures of more than 200 mm H_2O cannot be maintained for a long period without transudation. In patients suffering from Eustachian tube dysfunction without inflammation, it must be stressed that active opening of the tube (swallowing, yawning, mastication) is not completely effective. In normal individuals, it does not even occur 50% of the time, but does occur sufficiently to reduce the negative pressure in stages. This explains how chronic negative pressure may be set up, insufficient to cause exudation or transudation, but continuing over a long enough period to retract a weakened tympanic membrane.

The suction-insufflation theory of the Eustachian tube (Van Dishoek) is illustrated perfectly here: two synergic forces push air from the nasopharynx towards the middle ear – increased pressure in the pharynx produced by swallowing and suction caused by a previously created negative pressure in the middle ear. In 1971, Elnar et al. [63] noticed that the volume of air entering the middle ear is smaller when the negative pressure is higher – there is suction of the cartilaginous tube which reduces its lumen.

The mobility of the tympanic membrane is undoubtedly important in equalizing the pressure, since it can be moved by only a very slight change in pressure and this can compensate for a relatively large variation in volume. In the same year, Elnar et al. [63] also showed that it is easier for the tympanic membrane to equalize increased pressure than decreased pressure. For the same reason, when the tympanic membrane is weakened and/or distended, and even when the Eustachian tube has regained a proper active opening tonus, the membrane will tend to stick to the incudostapedial area or the promontory. In this sense, some authors have spoken of 'pulsion phenomena' in the pathology of retraction pockets; the least negative pressure in the tympanic cavity, even within normal physiological limits, will give rise to change of volume which will be all the greater if the tympanic membrane is weakened. This leads us to the idea of chronic hypoventilation.

Volumetric Properties of the Tympanic Cavity and the Mastoid

In 1959, Shambaugh compared the tympanic cavity and the mastoid to a miniature lung in which the larynx and the trachea are represented by the Eustachian tube. This is undoubtedly an idea which gives food for thought, the main difference being that the tympanic membrane can compensate for variations in volume. The air content of the mastoid has a close relationship with its mucosa and the two closely linked functions are related to the acoustic and volumetric properties. Both are often neglected, as Austin [14] has pointed out, while too much attention is given to the Eustachian tube and the ossicular chain. The tympanic membrane itself regulates pressure [105] by means of its elastic fibres which are missing in cases of atelectasis or retraction pockets, and which are either missing or abnormal after tympanoplasty. This is why homografts give the most satisfactory results from a functional point of view. Changes in the mobility and the elasticity of the tympanic membrane make it less able to incite the opening of the Eustachian tube because of the disappearance of its proprioceptive reflex. The middle ear cavities are very sensitive to partial variations in pressure. We are thus led to consider the possibility that there may be functional disturbances in gas exchanges in the mucosa, either linked to the constitution of the mucosa, or caused by disease. Eden [59] showed that both the sympathetic receptors (caroticotympanic branch) and parasympathetic receptors (glomic cells, paratympanic plexus) are sensitive to changes in quality and quantity of the gases in the tympanic and mastoid cavities, and can act on the velotubal muscles by reflex arc. We cannot mention pressure without mentioning volume, and we cannot mention volume in the mastoid without mentioning the development of the pneumatization of the mastoid. This begins in the fetus. The mastoid cell system is formed before it is aerated. The volume may keep on increasing until after puberty, initially by the resorption of the embryonic mesenchyme and later by extension of the cell system. Why is the mastoid so often sclerotic or eburnated in patients with chronic otitis media and cholesteatoma? Since the beginning of the century, researchers have pursued either the genetic or the environmentalist theory.

Genetic Theory

Cheatle, followed by Diamant and Diamant [57] hold the view that the degree of pneumatization of the mastoid, which varies from one individual to another, follows a Gaussian curve. It has even been claimed that these authors regarded the lack of mastoid cells as a cause of chronic disease – which only goes to show how difficult it is to make oneself understood despite clearly expressing oneself. Our thorough study of their work has led us to conclude that the claim was not an accurate interpretation. Diamant and Diamant gave their position as the following:

(a) Even a very highly sclerotic mastoid may be found with an anatomically and functionally normal middle ear;

(b) But when unilateral otitis media occurs in a patient, it always affects the less pneumatized ear, wherever the perforation may be. Normally, in any given individual, the difference between the pneumatization of the two ears never exceeds a certain statistical coefficient (approximately 20% of the surface of the more highly pneumatized ear);

(c) There is a marked difference between paracentral and postero-superior perforations. The statistical distribution of pneumatization follows a Gaussian curve in the former case and a hyperbolic curve in the latter case;

(d) Cholesteatoma is a clinical entity upon which Diamant and Diamant's approach can throw no particular light. Compact mastoids predominate, which is easily understandable since marginal perforations are often caused by cholesteatoma, which can nonetheless appear on highly pneumatized mastoids. Our epidemiological knowledge has expanded greatly since Diamant and Diamant's research (prior to 1952). In particular, we know that more or less prolonged and totally unsuspected seromucous effusion affects 30% of the population up to the age of 18 months, and 10% up to the age of 5 years. This does not perhaps change the Gaussian distribution, but would in our view justify new research on a sample population whose normality would be judged by strict, modern otoscopic, audiometric and impedance metric criteria. Albrecht in 1925 and Schwartz [199] in 1944, predecessors of Plester [167, 168] at Tübingen, looked more closely at the purely hereditary factor by comparing 59 pairs of monozygotic and 35 pairs of dizygotic twins. There is a highly significant relationship between monozygotic twins on the one hand, and parents and children on the other hand. Schwartz showed, on several family trees, how the hereditary transmission of reduced pneumatization (which appears to be relatively dominant) is related to the appearance of an invagination or an attic cholesteatoma. It is obviously not possible to say which (the dense mastoid or the invagination of the pars flaccida) is hereditary, or which causes the other. In fact, both may depend on a third parameter, more important from the pathogenic point of view. Ultersdorf and Plester [168] have found a significant and close statistical relationship between the angle of the clivus and the extent of pneumatization. These authors think that the phylogenetic evolution of the Eustachian tube, which is round and wide in animals but oval and narrow in humans, depends on the evolution of the shape of the base of the cranium. In humans, the upright posture has led to deformations which explain the characteristic anatomy of the Eustachian tube. The most important genetic parameter would thus appear to be a predisposition to tubal dysfunction, although we can go no further than this.

The importance of family factors in chronic inflammation of the middle ear is a well-established epidemiological notion, but it is impossible to say why the disease develops, or does not develop, into cholesteatoma. Some authors have attributed it to an ethnic predisposition, remarking on the fact that Eskimos and Australian Aborigines, who are often affected by chronic otitis media, have fewer cholesteatomas than the white population. For black Americans, Harell [102] gives a percentage of cholesteatomas which is comparable to the percentage of white Americans, although the incidence of otitis in general is much higher in the white population.

Environmentalist Theory

In 1918, Wittmaack claimed that a compact mastoid was always pathological, and that there was a significant relationship between this and attic retraction. In his view, the anatomical condition was due to inadequate trophicity of the mucosa of the tympanic cavity and Eustachian tube. He related the development of the cell system to the histological characteristics of the mucosa of the middle ear, which he divided into three types – hypo-, normo- or hyperplastic – each of which favoured the development of pneumatization to a different extent. This was purely a theoretical proposition, based on a small number of histological samples taken from cadavers. In 1927, Alexander claimed that Wittmaack's work was totally unscientific, and stressed that the three types of mucosa could be found together in the same specimen, and that any distinction between the three was difficult to make and necessarily subjective. In 1937, Wittmaack himself denied the existence of any correlation between the type of mucosa and cell development.

In 1959, Tumarkin [244] again raised the standard of the environmentalist theory with a strong attack on Diamant and Diamant's opinion. His main argument was based on a comparison between the degree of pneumatization in two selected populations, one from the working-class districts of Liverpool, and the other from a richer background. Planimetry showed an average of 9.7 cm^2 for the former group, and 13.54 cm^2 for the latter. Furthermore, since the disease was more common in adults, he accepted that younger generations might have benefitted from medical progress and from a general improvement in standards of hygiene and diet.

Ueda and Eguchi [cf. 186] compared pneumatization in two populations, one from the period before the introduction of antibiotics (1936–1942), and the other from the period when the use of antibiotics was expanding rapidly (1948–1952). They found no difference in the extent of pneumatization between the two periods. It is in fact inaccurate to refer to the environment as a whole, since it includes a multitude of different factors, Kolihova et al. [123] carried out a longitudinal study of the radiological planimetry of the mastoids of children affected by bouts of acute otitis. They found that, after treatment, pneumatization started developing again, and attained near-average figures. These authors are therefore of the opinion that middle ear infection slows down pneumatization.

The pathology of the middle ear in patients with cleft palates is interesting because of its high frequency [252]. Severeid [200] has shown that the duration of acute or subacute conditions depends, for this particular section of the population, on the age at which the condition first appears – average duration of more than 10 years with age at onset of less than 3 months, and duration of 5 years when age at onset of otitis was around 9 months. In the latter group, the surface of the mastoid was between 6 and 11 cm^2, and in the former less than 6 cm^2. Patients who developed cholesteatomas had mastoids of less than 3 cm^2. The pneumatization of mastoid is thus reduced by the duration of inflammation of the tympanic cavity and Eustachian tube, and/or by its early onset. The risk of complications (including cholesteatoma) is increased when the mastoid is less pneumatized. It is difficult to state with certainty that Eustachian tube dysfunction is the essential characteristic of the ear in individuals with cleft palates. The modifications in local and regional embryonal induction may have other implications, such as the quality of the reactions of the mucosa or the connective tissue to inflammation.

We know little of the development of ossification centres in the mastoid, and individual variations in bone metabolism are difficult to analyse. Andreasson has shown that there is no absolute correlation between the planimetric surface and the volume of the tympanic and mastoid cavities, and the unreliability of radiological criteria is well known. This unreliability is confirmed daily by radioclinical comparisons during surgery. Must we go into the old argument again? For Heine [cf. 28], compact mastoids were the result of chronic suppuration, while in Cheatle's opinion the infection only became chronic when the mastoid was sclerotic. Longitudinal studies of each case and comparisons between healthy ears and the controlateral diseased ears are of greater value than statistical studies of large groups. It is undoubtedly true that a mastoid may become sclerotic as a result of repeated infection and/or prolonged dysfunction of the Eustachian tube. This is why Friedman [82] makes a distinction between (a) a primary sclerotic mastoid which consists largely of diploë and in which the Haversian system is present, even in the sclerotic zones, and (b) a secondary sclerotic mastoid, which is characterized by compact, layered or trabecular bone made up of successive layers. The density varies from layer to layer, which is emphasized by the presence of rows of osteoblasts at the beginning of their formation. Areas of osteoclastic activity are often found at the edge of progressive lesions.

Hermann and Riehm [cf. 82] proposed the adoption, depending on the degree of difficulty of histological interpretation, of the distance between the lateral sinus and the posterior canal wall as a distinguishing criterion. This distance is short in a constitutionally compact mastoid. Such research into the pneumatization and the volume of the mastoid, as Diamant and Diamant [57] indeed point out, throws little light on the question of cholesteatoma. They provide a factual basis for a certain number of interesting ideas which the surgeon will take into account in his analysis of the indication for surgery. In brief:

(a) A normal mastoid should be adequately pneumatized. The degree of pneumatization is more dependent on the proper functioning of the Eustachian tube than directly on genetic factors, but Eustachian tube function is itself dependent on genetic factors.

(b) The best standard by which to assess the pneumatization of a mastoid is to compare it with the opposite ear (provided that it is healthy).

(c) The reduction of pneumatization in chronic otitis media depends on the age at which inflammatory phenomena first appear and on the severity and duration. After a mastoidectomy for severe lesions in children, pneumatization may start developing again.

(d) Research into pneumatization is valid insofar as the volume of the tympanic and mastoid cavities is free, when there is a certain correlation between volume and surface, and radiological contrasts are generally clear and easily read. This was the case for Diamant and Diamant's research which compared central and posterosuperior perforations.

(e) Cholesteatoma is a very special problem. A cholesteatoma involves a variable amount of space and gives rise to bony reactions which develop slowly and over a long period, with the association of bone resorption and bone construction. Sclerosis or eburnation of the mastoid is generally neither hereditary, congenital, nor secondary to childhood otitis. It is the result of a very long process, a defence mechanism which tends to limit the pathological process to the antrum [87].

Therefore, it is not immaterial to note the type of mastoid in which a cholesteatoma is developing – an initially eburnated type, or the type that will become more dense on contact with the cholesteatoma. Radiological pictures of compact mastoids can be particularly misleading – the thickness of the outer cortex makes it impossible to assess the deep pneumatization and its irregularities. These are what Steufer [cf. 248] calls 'dangerous mastoids' which may hold surprises in store for the surgeon. The free space in the tympanic and mastoid cavities varies from one individual to the next. According to Silberger [cf. 186], average volumes are: (a) 12.2 ml in a normal ear; (b) 3.47 ml when there is a central perforation, and (c) 2.64 ml when there is a marginal perforation.

This idea of 'free volume' brings us back more or less to Diamant and Diamant's [57] studies, in that they may lead the surgeon to create a large mastoid cavity in order to improve or normalize the volumetric aspect. The work of Elnar et al. [63] was an attempt to clarify this subject pragmatically. They confirmed the research of Rin et al. [177], showing that the volume of gas absorbed daily in the mastoid cavity does not depend on the volume of the cavity – it remains steady at 0.80 ml/24 h. Negative pressure therefore develops more rapidly in smaller cavities. When considering the radiological assessment, which does not in any case give a true picture, it must be remembered that congestion of the mucosa increases the rate of gaseous exchange and that its thickening markedly reduces the apparent volume of the cavities. This is therefore an unstable system, the physiological balance of which may quickly become decompensated, giving rise to rapidly irreversible lesions. Although many factors are involved and this research needs to be confirmed, Smyth [219] suggests that the role of the tympanomastoid volume is significant when series of tympanoplasties with mas-

toidectomy are compared to series without. In reality the most important role, besides the proper function of the Eustachian tube, seems to
be played by the quality of the mucosa of the tympanic cavity and
Eustachian tube, with all the unknown factors that this implies. From
both the functional and the morphological point of view, the future of
a closed-technique and even of an open-technique tympanoplasty is
essentially linked, disregarding for the moment any possibility of a residual cholesteatoma, to the way in which all the middle ear cavities
are aerated and lined. The existence of prolonged negative pressure in
the middle ear seeems to be an important factor, the importance of
which is felt stressed by all the authors. There is a tendency to lay the
blame on a standard-type obstruction, going from the ear to the nasopharynx, with a slow and prolonged build-up of negative pressure and
a poor ability to equalize pressures during functional tests. The idea of
'dyspatency' should be replaced by that of 'dysfunction', since air may
also pass from the middle ear to the nasopharynx, thus modifying the
volumetric properties of the functional unit composed of the Eustachian tube, the middle ear, the tympanic membrane and the mastoid
cavities. The Eustachian tube is closed when at rest, which explains (a)
why it opens when the pressure gradient is positive in the middle ear,
and (b) why it becomes blocked when the pressure gradient is negative
in the middle ear, with excess pressure in the nasopharynx and external auditory meatus. Active opening of the Eustachian tube can only
be effective within certain limits – that it may be forced open by a
negative pressure gradient towards the nasopharynx as is the case in
sniffing and snoring, during which the air in the middle ear may be
sucked, violently and repeatedly, into the cavum. The negative pressure applied may reach, and even exceed, 1,000 mm H_2O [134].

It is difficult for the present to be sure what mechanism is involved
in this abnormal patency of the Eustachian tube from the nasopharynx
to the ear – increase in the rigidity of the walls of the tube, excessive
muscle relaxation, a valve phenomenon in the mucosa, or others may
be involved. Eustachian tube dysfunction must be considered in its
widest sense. Besides the classically accepted role of the tubal muscles,
Tomoda et al. [236] recently demonstrated the elastic and collagen fi-
brillary texture around the Eustachian tube mucosa. They describe:

(1) An internal elastic layer clinging tightly to the basement membrane of the epithelium of the Eustachian tube at its pharyngeal orifice. In the middle part of the cartilaginous tube, and near the isthmus,

this elastic layer is only present in the floor and lateral wall of the Eustachian tube. It is very thin in children and is also more elastic in adults. It may explain why the pharyngeal portion of the tube is so little affected by yawning or swallowing. Both these phenomena have a particular effect on the middle portion and the isthmus, especially in children;

(2) A circular collagen layer in the middle portion, which explains the permanence of the shape of the nasopharynx. At this point it is in fact clearly separated from the external layer;

(3) A longitudinal collagen layer, made up of fibres surrounding the whole Eustachian tube and cling closely to the previous layer in the middle portion and around the isthmus. The number of collagen fibres increases with age. Tomoda et al. suggest that this elastic and collagenous system: (a) provides a certain resistance to outside pressures; (b) maintains a certain degree of tension which returns the lumen of the Eustachian tube to its relaxed dimensions after contraction of the tensor veli palatini muscle, and (c) makes it possible to coordinate an associated slide rotation movement of the cartilage in relation to the lumen of the tube during muscle contractions.

The full value of these anatomical observations is brought out by the manometric measurements carried out by Magnuson [137] who stresses that clinical assessment of Eustachian tube function is quite inadequate, since it amounts, apart from forced insufflation, to the assessment of the ability to equalize pressure during swallowing. A certain number of surveys have shown that high negative pressure can appear in atelectasic ears even in spite of a relatively adequate ability to equalize pressure. Magnuson [136] stresses the degree of negative pressure (up to 1,000 mm H_2O) which can be induced by sniffing or any form of breathing acting on increased nasal or nasopharyngeal impedance (collapse of the nasal valve on inspiration, hypertrophy of the adenoids, frequent rhinitis). He also shows that there is no strict parallel between a poor ability to equalize pressure and the ability to set up a high negative pressure in the tympanic cavity. Any combination of the two is possible and a thorough examination of each patient, repeated over a period, must be made in order to assess Eustachian tube dysfunction: from a dynamic viewpoint, one should understand this method of assessment today, without losing sight of the complexity of the movements and anatomical structures of the Eustachian tube.

Falk [65] has confirmed the validity of this remark in a survey of two groups of patients with cleft palates, all of whom suffered from inadequate patency of Eustachian tube, materialized by a decrease in the ability to equalize negative pressures: (a) The first group (29 ears) showed recurrent mucous effusion without tympanic retraction. By sniffing, 7% of these patients could induce a stable negative pressure ($\times 170$ mm H_2O). (b) The second group (20 ears) showed clear signs of tympanic retraction (atelectatic ears with or without cholesteatoma). This group had the same difficulty as the other in equalizing applied negative pressures, but 65% of them could induce a negative pressure ($\times 230$ mm H_2O) by sniffing. The variation was from 120 to 500 mm H_2O for this group. Furthermore, one third of these patients were habitual sniffers. Magnuson [135] was recently able to study a group of patients who had undergone closed-technique surgery and had developed postoperative problems (especially retraction pockets). In his opinion, the essential factor in these postoperative problems is not so much a poor ability to equalize pressures, but rather an ability to induce high negative pressures, by sniffing for example.

Magnuson suggests that a routine examination should be made to determine whether a patient has this ability to induce high negative pressures, and that this should be taken into account when considering the indications for surgery. Koch and Straehler-Pohl [122] confirm, in a survey of 55 patients who had undergone closed-technique surgery, that the development of a new epitympanic invagination in 27 cases, up to 5 or 6 years later, is unconnected with the ability to equalize pressures. The classical view is to consider obstruction of the Eustachian tube as the primordial factor in the pathogenesis of chronic inflammatory conditions of the middle ear, causing negative pressure by gas resorption, will all the consequences to which such negative pressure leads. Thorough study of chronic seromucous otitis media [19, 20, 31] has shown that there is no true mechanical obstruction, even when the threshold for passive opening of the tube is high. On the contrary, in many cases the Eustachian tube is open, or opens too readily. In fact, the dilemma, from a functional point of view, is on the one hand to isolate the middle ear from the cavum, and on the other to ensure sufficient aeration for the metabolism of the mucosa. In physiological conditions, the Eustachian tube is closed and only opens intermittently. It is greatly to the credit of Magnuson and Falk that they have shown many Eustachian tubes which are incapable of remaining passively closed when at rest. Besides the exaggerated clinical picture of a widely open Eustachian tube, there are minor, long-lasting dysfunctions which the patients (especially children) find difficult to analyse, and our usual audiometric methods are inadequate to assess and quantify these problems. The subjective symptoms caused by this dysfunction vary from one moment to the next, or from one day to the next, in the same patient – difficulty in opening may alternate with inability to close the tube depending on the meteorological conditions, or on the inflammation of the nasopharynx. When the Eustachian tube does not close properly, sniffing becomes a reflex in order to reduce autophonia and/or deafness. This is why many children become habitual sniffers without obvious explanations. There is a tendency for sniffing to produce long-term transmission deafness and high negative pressure than Eustachian tube obstruction.

Sniffing has little effect when the tympanic membrane is intact or firm, but it will aggravate the retraction of a weakened and slack membrane. Some patients become very fussy about their Eustachian tubes, and find it difficult to understand why sniffing sometimes relieves and sometimes worsens their functional problems. When the tympanic membrane is completely atelectatic, or when there is a fixed retraction pocket, manoeuvres of the Eustachian tube have little effect on the functional symptoms, and tubal dysfunction persists, with all its unwelcome effects on the anatomical structures. It is all the more true that, when a cholesteatoma is present, the subjective symptoms of the inadequate closing of the Eustachian tube disappear, while the deleterious effects of the negative pressure persist. In Magnuson's view, this is the most likely explanation for retraction pockets and recurrences after closed-technique cholesteatectomy. It must be made clear exactly what is meant by the term 'sniffing'. In addition to the obvious, socially undesirable sniff, many patients develop high negative pressure in the cavum when there is nasal obstruction due to rhinitis, or by breathing in deeply with even a slight collapse of the nasal valve. The dogmatic hostility of paediatricians towards tonsillectomy means that we can now see children with highly hypertrophied tonsils, and their consequences on the heart have been described in the literature on the subject. When the patient is in a reclining position, during sleep, these enormous tonsils fall backwards, leading to a reduction of free space, which in turn causes considerable worsening of the negative pressure in the nasopharynx. The following may serve as an outline to explain the development of the condition in the majority of cases:

(a) Inflammatory phenomena develop behind a closed tympanic membrane more or less independently of any obstruction, or inadequate passive closing, of the Eustachian tube. It would appear that inadequate patency of the Eustachian tube is important at this stage. It is at least as often secondary to these phenomena as it is primary.

(b) These phenomena vary from one day to the next, and from season to season, with a spontaneous tendency to improve over the year. The future evolution of the ear is determined in childhood.

(c) These inflammatory phenomena may vary in severity and duration. They give rise to enzymatic reactions which may cause irreversible lesions of the collagen tissue. Some studies have shown that atrophy of the tympanic membrane, or the disappearance or rupture of the collagen fibres, is due more to histochemical phenomena than to the degree of negative pressure. The compliance of the tympanic membrane thus increases gradually. It may be supposed by Tomoda et al. [236] that the collagen tissue surrounding the tissue of the Eustachian tube is subject to comparable changes. Inadequate closing of the tube could be explained by changes in the structures supporting the mucosa. There is a gradual progression from inadequate patency to tubal dysfunction. Sniffing, which has little effect as long as the tympanic membrane is intact, may contribute to its stretching when the membrane responds more and more to the negative pressure. The accumulation of epithelial squamae, and infection from outside, exercise maximum influence in such cases.

The Idea of a Precursor of Cholesteatoma

The main interest in taking a systemic approach to the aetiopathogenic factors in cholesteatoma is to bring out the idea of a precursor of cholesteatoma. When there is epithelial invasion of the tympanic cavity and the mastoid, whether this be: (a) by a sac cholesteatoma, the classical pearly tumour; (b) or by complete epithelialization, or a retraction pocket filled with debris; (c) or by a disorganized epidermosis, then the pathology is 'under way' and will continue inexorably at its own speed, which will vary from case to case. Only one therapeutic approach can be adopted – surgery, whether using an open or a closed technique, or a variant of either.

All forms of cholesteatoma can damage the anatomical structure, and in the long term the function of the ear. If we wish to prevent cholesteatoma, it is essential that we know what anatomico-clinical conditions can lead to its formation. Is this possible, either in full or in part? Can we define attitudes of 'active surveillance' in order to stabilize some of these conditions? Is it possible to adopt a pragmatic and/or empirical attitude with some degree of effectiveness even though we are not fully aware of all the details of the mechanisms involved in the formation of cholesteatomas? And even if we do not know what all these mechanisms are, can we act on some of them before the condition becomes irreversible? Analytic reasoning tends to give priority to certain factors: (a) at the First International Conference on Cholesteatoma in Iowa, inflammatory and enzymatic phenomena were in vogue, and (b) at the Second International Conference on Cholesteatoma at Tel Aviv, the idea of Eustachian tube dysfunction and negative pressure was to the fore.

In Sheehy's view, Eustachian tube problems are not obvious and the behaviour of the mucosa is predominant. He does not, however, treat cholesteatoma differently in children and in adults. It is true that his opinion is not shared by all authors. It is obvious that inflammatory phenomena are more important, and infection coming from the Eustachian tube more frequent, in children, while infection from outside is the distinguishing feature for some neglectful adults. Embryonic induction is still important in the child's pretympanic and tympanic membrane, and desquamation is more easily activated by inflammatory phenomena. These phenomena will no doubt be stressed at a Third International Conference on Cholesteatoma. What conditions can we, at the present time, consider to be precursors of cholesteatoma?

In the attic:
(1) Retraction;
(2) Epithelial migration disorders;
(3) The accumulation of debris;
(4) Scabs;
(5) Infection;
(6) Proliferation of connective tissue;
(7) Bone resorption with a spontaneous atticotomy which is not retentive but is likely to become so;
(8) Closure of the angle between the pars flaccida and the meatus.

Although it is not possible to be certain of the aetiology of minor anomalies in the region of the pars flaccida, the following data must be taken into account: (a) The frequently constitutional nature of depressions of the pars flaccida and the narrowness of the angle formed between it and the meatus. Schwartz demonstrated that this is a feature which runs in families. (b) Individual, secondary or acquired variability of the connective tissue which here separates the squamous epithelium from the mucosa. Marx [cf. 28] showed that it is slack, practically nonexistent in 50% of cases, and this has been confirmed by one of the present authors and Marquet [139, 140]. (c) The frequency with which a sclerotic mastoid coexists with a retraction of the pars flaccida – more often than with lesions of the pars tensa.

Alongside medical action on the Eustachian tube, surveillance of these otoscopic aspects must be accompanied by dry cleaning under the microscope, avoiding any maceration, and the recommendation of alcohol or slightly acid baths. Meticulous thoroughness in cleaning these lesions may be a true preventive approach. In Goodhill's [98] opinion, prophylaxis may go as far as strengthening the pars flaccida with perichondrium or tragus cartilage.

In the pars tensa:

(1) An unfixed retraction pocket;

(2) A retraction pocket fixed to the incudostapedial joint;

(3) A retraction pocket fixed in the posterior part of the mesotympanum;

(4) Epithelial migration disorders and even the slightest accumulation of debris on the surface of the tympanic membrane;

(5) Maceration and infection or some aspects of myringitis;

(6) The appearance of granulomas through rupture of the epithelium (a) on the bone (bony sulcus or ossicles); (b) on the floor of the tympanic cavity, or (c) on the annulus;

(7) Bone resorption, most frequently in the medial posterosuperior region of the meatus. It is often difficult to reconstitute the chain of causation of the otoscopic aspects for each particular case. In the vast majority of cases, they follow a retrotympanic seromucous effusion which has passed unnoticed. We know that between 20 and 25% of cases of seromucous otitis present therapeutic problems because of recurrence or slow development, but very few of them turn into cholesteatomas while under clinical observation. The patient often seeks medical advice again a few years later, after an interval with no clear

clinical signs, when he has fully developed cholesteatoma. In this case the explanation may be that after the liquid inflammatory reactions in the tympanic cavity have disappeared, the accumulation of desquamated cells may make the transition to cholesteatoma more likely in certain conditions. There is no doubt that, given the same conditions, a cholesteatoma will not develop in every ear. One example appears to be demonstrative in this connection: the exceptional rarity of cholesteatoma in a patient operated on for otosclerosis, even when he has had too large an atticotomy with a retraction pocket;

(8) The rarity with which fenestration cavities for otosclerosis were affected by true cholesteatoma although they often became infected; the greater frequency, on the other hand, with which so-called drainage atticoantrotomies, or the old anteroposterior techniques 'as required by the lesions', developed iatrogenic cholesteatoma over the years. The existence of a negative pressure, which is high sometimes, is shown in the majority of ears with retraction pockets or cholesteatoma. This was as much as – 500 mm H_2O in 10 observations out of a series of 52 cases studied by Holmquist and Lindeman [105].

It is true that a high negative pressure may persist in the middle ear for a long period without developing into a cholesteatoma. It is relatively difficult to give definite criteria on what constitutes a precursor of cholesteatoma, and not all retraction pockets can be put into this category. The 'danger' criteria are: (a) the rupture of the pocket; (b) the adhesion of the pocket to the incudostapedial region, which seems to favour and activate the proliferation of epithelium, and (c) the depth of the pocket and of its possible digitations into the mucosal folds and ligaments and around the ossicles, which favour the retention of epithelial debris.

The loss of the self-cleansing ability for epithelial debris is the common factor in all the precursors of cholesteatoma, and it is probably the most important function of the tympanic membrane. Eliachar and Joachims [62] stress the fact that durable ventilation of the middle ear by an aeration tube may partially reverse or stabilize the process of accumulation of squamous debris. Buckingham [29] is of the same opinion. This might, if it cannot actually avoid the need for major surgery, provide the best possible conditions for the repair of the ear, both from the anatomical and the functional point of view.

With this in mind, Sade et al. [188] have suggested a classification of retraction pockets which could serve as a guide to the indications for treatment. As a practical level, when one of these precursors of cholesteatoma is observed, a certain number of steps should be taken: (a) regular inspection and follow-up, without interruption, even if everything seems to be satisfactory; (b) cleaning under the microscope; (c) no penetration of water into the meatus (absolutely essential); (d) spa treatment and physiotherapy for the Eustachian tube, within an overall context of respiratory re-education; (e) treatment to modify any other illnesses, and finally, (f) surgery to strengthen the tympanic membrane with perichondrium or thinned cartilage. It must never, however, be thought that the results of such surgery are necessarily definitive.

Clinical Evaluation

The diagnosis of cholesteatoma is generally easy. It is helped nowadays by the systematic use of the binocular microscope in the consulting room. A valuable aid, thanks to the considerable progress which has been made in this field, is radiology.

Circumstances in Which Cholesteatoma Is Detected

Schematically, it may be said that the specialist can be led to diagnose cholesteatoma in five types of situation: (1) examination for purulent otorrhoea; (2) examination for deafness; (3) occurrence of a complication; (4) routine ENT examination, and (5) detection during an operation. The relative frequencies of the different sets of circumstances in which cholesteatoma is detected have recently been established by Chuard [45] in a computer-assisted study which is summarized in table I.

Purulent Otorrhoea

Purulent otorrhoea is a common symptom of chronic otitis. Patients often put up with it for many years. It is never painful. Habit, lack of information or fear of surgery are all factors which may explain neglect over a long period. Neglect is even encouraged in some areas by the popular tradition that otorrhoea is a necessary evil: 'It's just the poison finding a way out' or 'It's a cold in the ear!' The otorrhoea of cholesteatoma, which is a sign of infection, is, however, distinguishable from the otorrhoea of simple chronic suppurative otitis media – by its fetid nature which may even offend others in the vicinity and by its continuous evolution, which may occasionally be intermitent, but is generally independent of rhinopharyngitis. Despite proper treatment of the affected area, and strict hygiene, including cleaning of the meatus, avoiding bathing and splashes of water when washing, it persists and does not lose its fetid odor.

Table I. Circumstances in which cholesteatoma is detected (from a computer-assisted study of 1,071 cases of cholesteatoma over a period of 10 years)

	Number of cases	%
Purulent otorrhoea	571	53
Deafness	183	17
Complication		
Vertigo	81	8
Polyp	52	
Tinnitus	17	
Pain	6	
Mastoiditis	5	
Facial paralysis	5	
Labyrinthitis	3	
Meningitis	2	
Intracranial abscess	2	
Various	24	
Operation	4	
Trauma	4	
Routine examination	92	9
Recurrence	20	

Bleeding from the Ear

The spontaneous appearance of a blood-stained discharge from the meatus is an occurrence which has the advantage of alarming the patient and causing him to seek medical advice. It is not a frequent event. The amount of blood involved is never serious. It is the result of bleeding from polyps or granular mucous membrane. It is thus a sign of infection.

Deafness

It is not exceptional for the hearing to remain normal, or only slightly impaired, during a large part of the evolution of a cholesteatoma; because the ossicular chain is intact, or because the cholesteatoma itself achieves the columellar effect, or because retraction of the tympanic membrane has resulted in spontaneous tympanoplasty. In the majority of cases, however, the hearing is impaired. The deafness experienced by each patient is nonetheless extremely variable, willingly tolerated if the lesion is unilateral, but soon becoming troublesome if both ears are affected. Since the improvement in the reputation of ear surgery over the last few years, deafness is not uncommonly the first functional sign which leads the patient to seek medical advice. For the same degree of deafness, the inconvenience experienced varies greatly from one individual to another, depending on his or her social or intellectual level, professional obligations or need to communicate. There is no interrelation between the size of the cholesteatoma and the degree to which hearing is impaired. Deafness may precede the appearance of the cholesteatoma, especially in a case where there is a predisposition to defective aeration of the middle ear, Eustachian tube dysfunction, or serous or mucous otitis media.

Tinnitus

Tinnitus is, in some cases, the major functional symptom leading a patient to seek medical advice. Sensations of fullness or a blocked ear, or popping noises, may be grouped under the same head.

Vertigo

The occurrence of rotatory vertigo or imbalance in a case of chronic otitis media points to the possible presence of a fistula in the labyrinth as a result of cholesteatoma. There may be more pronounced vertigo, immobilizing the patient for several days, with a risk of being interpreted as Ménière's disease. It must be hoped that at this stage the symptom will draw the doctor's attention to the ear. If this vertigo can be reproduced by applying pressure to the tragus or the mastoid with a wool-carrier or Siegle's speculum, it is the 'fistula sign' which is almost pathognomonic of cholesteatoma.

Facial Paralysis

Facial paralysis as a complication of cholesteatoma may be partial or total, sudden or progressive. It is rarely the first symptom. Hemispasm, which is exceptional, may have the same diagnostic significance.

Infection

Infection may result in localized pain in the mastoid region, in headaches in the temporal region, fever and sometimes, paradoxically, in the drying up of a purulent otorrhoea for several days. All these symptoms are often alleviated, and then disappear, as the otorrhoea returns, draining the ear. On the other hand, infection may develop a true mastoiditis: with violent pains, redness and oedema in the mastoid region, which is painful to pressure. One important feature distinguishes it from otitis media – the painless immobilization of the auricle. Emergency surgery makes it possible to detect a cholesteatoma which may be either still intracavitary or already developing outwards to the external cortex. It is advisable to make a systematic search for any signs of an associated intracranial complication which may be developing unseen during this bout of infection.

Intracranial Complications

The ENT specialist called in as a consultant by the neurology, neurosurgery or infectious diseases department may be led to diagnose cholesteatoma in a patient with meningitis, a cerebral or cerebellar abscess, or thrombophlebitis of the lateral sinus.

Systematic Examination

The development of the cholesteatoma may for a long time present few or no symptoms. It is now often treated at an increasingly early stage, thanks to the increase in the number of routine examinations, e.g., at school, during medical inspection, on joining the armed forces, in the course of general health check-ups, and to the incrasingly widespread use of the binocular microscope by the ENT consultant.

Detection During an Operation

In a not inconsiderable number of cases, cholesteatoma is discovered during an operation. This is the case: (a) for the majority of intact tympanic membrane cholesteatomas; (b) for certain attic retraction pockets which have been recognized, but whose extent can only be appreciated during the course of the operation; (c) for certain tympanosclerosis, infiltration of the remaining part of the tympanic membrane favouring and concealing epidermic migration to its internal surface; (d) for certain cases of chronic otitis media which appear simple but in which epidermic invaginations, because of their situation (facial recess, tympanic sinus, hypotympanum), are completely hidden from otoscopic examination.

It is clear that the surgeon must be extremely prudent and vigilant, both in his clinical examination and in surgical action.

Positive Diagnosis

Positive diagnosis of cholesteatoma of the middle ear is made, primarily, by otoscopy; paraclinical examinations (radiological, audiometric and bacteriological) and general ENT examination each provide additional information which will be discussed.

Otoscopic Examination

Diagnosis of cholesteatoma is based on the detection of one pathognomonic sign: the presence of stratified squamous epithelium which has accumulated in the middle ear.

Technique

Otoscopic examination must be carried out according to strict rules.

Binocular Microscope. The clinical use of the microscope has become compulsory in otology. The otoscopic examination benefits in three ways: (1) *Proper Illumination:* the incidence of the light is almost identical with that of the visual image. With the diffusion of the light, no zone is left shadow. (2) *Binocular vision:* the traditional examination using a mirror only allows monocular vision. Certain optical effects or superimpositions may lead to mistaken interpretation. The microscope makes it possible to distinguish even the slightest relief and to interpret the contour observed exactly. (3) *Magnification:* a magnification of 6×, or preferably 9×, is necessary and sufficient to identify the anatomical landmarks and pathological changes.

The combination of these three factors makes this examination practical to carry out and gives a welcome freedom of movement for cleaning, suction and palpation of the meatus and the tympanic cavity.

Instruments. Minimum requirements are: suction, and suckers with diameters varying from 0.5 to 2 mm; crocodile forceps, and a small blunt hook.

Position of the Patient. The patient's head lies on a headrest, the patient himself reclining on an examination table, arms extented along his body to favor a relaxed attitude. An examination can only be properly carried out if the patient is perfectly still, and the consultant must make every effort to win his confidence and allay his apprehension. It must be remembered that the ear is extremely sensitive and that the contact of an instrument with the external auditory meatus may be painful.

Position of the Consultant. He is seated on the same side as the ear being examined. His movements will be steadier if he rests the edge of his hand on the patient's head, controlling as far as possible his own movements and avoiding any incident should the patient move unexpectedly.

Methodology

Cleaning of the Meatus. The presence of cerumen and squamous debris in the external auditory meatus is physiological (and not the result of inadequate hygiene). It may be favoured by any underlying pathological condition. In the case of infection, the secretions are usually mixed with purulent waste matter and polypoid granulation. The otoscopic examination begins with the careful and nontraumatizing cleaning of the meatus, with the aid of suction, crocodile forceps and a blunt hook.

Anatomical Landmarks. The fibrous annulus is generally easy to locate. The short process of the malleus, an essential landmark, is sometimes more difficult to find. It must be identified to be used as a starting-point for the systematic exploration of the pars tensa and the pars flaccida.

Results

Diagnosis is Obvious. Examination of the middle ear reveals the cholesteatomatous debris which is characterized by: (a) its appearance, which is whitish, pearly, like cooked chestnut, or layered and squamous-like; (b) the fact that it responds easily to suction; (c) its lack of sensitivity; (d) its soft, friable and sometimes firm, fluctuant consistency, and (e) its lack of vascularization.

In a typical case, it comes from the attic, or from a posterosuperior marginal perforation. Infection may make it difficult to detect this characteristic appearance. It is indicated by two features which are themselves suggestive, namely otorrhoea and polyp. The otorrhoea is abundant, with a characteristically fetid odour, viscous, white or greenish coloured, and fills the meatus; it is necessary to use suction to uncover the lesions. The polyp (or granulations of variable size and number) is painless, red and congestive, and bleeds easily. It can be mobilized without difficulty by suction.

A large polyp blocking the external auditory meatus poses above all the problem of differential diagnosis, according to the aetiological circumstances: (a) in a young child (under 5 years) it should suggest the possibility of a sarcoma of the ear; (b) in an elderly patient, it may be a sign of the presence of a carcinoma. In this case it is often firmer and multilobed, and will bleed spontaneously, needing radiological and histological examinations. It is nonetheless true that in the majority of cases, it goes together with a cholesteatoma and requires surgical treatment.

It is generally easy to remove, either by suction or by gentle traction using the forceps. This makes it possible to see the fibrous annulus, localize the perforation and identify the cholesteatoma. Otherwise, the radiological and histological examinations will decide the therapeutic indications.

Diagnosis is Less Obvious. Widely varying clinical patterns may be observed, depending on: (a) the seat of the lesions: Schrapnell's membrane or pars flaccida, pars tensa, marginal or central; (b) their nature: retraction or perforation; (c) the inflammatory or cicatricial reaction (tympanosclerosis).

(a) Seat of the Lesions

Crust on Schrapnell's membrane: The discovery of a crust on the pars flaccida is in itself highly suspect. It must be prised up to reveal the cholesteatomatous matter. It is possible that the anatomic circumstances, sensitivity of the meatus or the presence of exostoses may make it impossible to remove. The clinical context is extremely important in such cases. The necessity for surgery is even more clearly indicated when there is a past history of infection, recurrent otorrhoea, a past history of polypectomy, a possibility of serous otitis, and unexplained conductive deafness. In such cases, a radiological examination is particularly useful for diagnosis.

Perforation of the pars tensa: In the typical case, the cholesteatoma is associated with a marginal posterosuperior perforation with destruction of the fibrous annulus. There are also cholesteatomas with central, nonmarginal anterosuperior and even anteroinferior perforations. These are often the most difficult cases.

(b) Nature of the Lesions

Certain forms of tympanic retraction are considered to be forerunners of cholesteatoma. There may be any one of the intermediate stages between ordinary epidermization and cholesteatoma. Such cases should be analyzed with three basic criteria in mind: (1) Mobility of the squamous membrane. Can the retracted membrane be detached from the subjacent surface? It is possible to use politzerization, the sucker and Siegle's speculum? Some authors suggest the use of nitrous oxide. (2) Collection of epidermal squames. Is the pocket the seat of intense or moderate desquamation? More important, is it self-cleansing or not? (3) Extent of the retraction pocket. The advantage of microscopic examination is to make it possible to explore in detail each fold of the pocket, and to draw attention to invaginations which escape the naked eye.

Depending on the topography, retraction pockets present different appearances under otoscopy:

(a) *Retraction of the pars flaccida:* It is often difficult to judge whether the appearances of the notch of Rivinus are pathological or normal. Failure to visualize the depths of a retraction pocket is highly suspicious and justifies surgical exploration which often reveals unexpected findings.

(b) *Retraction of the pars tensa:* Atrophy of the fibrous layer of the tympanum is the source of what is known as an atelectatic middle ear. The retraction may be: subligamentary, anterosuperior; anterior, rarely invaginating into the orifice of the Eustachian tube; inferior, lining the hypotympanic cells; posterior, lining the facial recess and the sinus tympani. Each of these areas may be the starting-point of a cholesteatoma of the inner or anterior parts of the attic or of the facial recess.

(c) Inflammatory or Cicatricial Reaction

Otitis externa: Inflammation of the skin of the meatus, with otorrhoea, obstruction causing deafness and sufficient pain on introducing the speculum to make it impossible to examine the tympanic membrane, make up the typical pattern shown by otitis externa. Otitis externa may be independent or it may be a complication of a concealed cholesteatoma. The diagnostic approach requires preliminary local and possibly general treatment. If diagnosis is still doubtful after this treatment, radiography may provide useful information: a perfectly pneumatized mastoid rules out the diagnosis of cholesteatoma in these precise circumstances; a characteristic picture of cholesteatoma may be present, with a sclerotic mastoid and widening of the antrum.

Chronic otitis media: If there is a large tympanic perforation, with the mucosa of the tympanic cavity being highly inflamed, a polypoid reaction, and mucopurulent otorrhoea, it may be difficult to determine the presence of epidermal debris. The presence of a polyp should always suggest a cholesteatoma. Very careful removal by suction causes bleeding which renders examination difficult and makes it necessary to see the patient again, after anti-inflammatory or anti-infectious treatment.

Tympanosclerosis: Tympanosclerosis presents particular difficulty. First, because of its appearance: a whitish formation, with a rounded, pearl-like shape, visible in the tympanic cavity or behind a tympanic membrane, is seen in both lesions. Palpation, when it is possible, removes the doubt – the pearl of cholesteatoma is soft, the plaque of tympanosclerosis is hard. Secondly, because of the possibility of association: according to Gristwood [99], it appears that tympanosclerosis is no more common in cases of cholesteatoma than in simple chronic otitis media. Major tympanosclerosis, on the other hand, leading the tympanic membrane and coating the walls of the tympanic cavity, guides the epidermis on the inner surface of the tympanum, in the hypotympanum and even in the anterior part of the attic or the orifice of the Eustachian tube, leading to the formation of cholesteatomas. It is to be remembered that one must be wary of such an association (a) because it is likely that the cholesteatoma will be much more difficult to recognize and (b) because the extent of the lesion may be great, favoured by a slow and silent development, without suppuration.

Diagnosis Is Difficult, or Even Impossible. Diagnosis may be difficult, or even impossible, because the pathognomonic sign, the presence of epidermal debris, is not visible on examination (a) because it is difficult to judge the extent of epidermic migration from the edges of a perforation; (b) or because the bony edge of the annulus hides an area where epidermization is suspected but which cannot be seen by otoscopic examination; it is necessary to use the possibilities provided by suction which can detach and bring to light hidden epidermic squama, or (c) because the cholesteatoma is developing behind a intact or healed tympanic membrane.

Texture of the tympanic membrane: Variations in the transparency of the tympanic membrane should be interpreted with caution. In certain cases, the texture makes it possible to observe a smooth-walled, white, regular, rounded, cystic formation behind the tympanic membrane, developing behind and in front of the handle of the malleus. This is the sac of the matrix of the cholesteatoma. Although this appearance is suggestive to a practised eye, it cannot be said to provide absolute proof. The extension of the sac may bring it into contact with the tympanic membrane, raise it, and make palpation possible, thus providing decisive information.

Discovery of cholesteatoma during myringotomy: Serous or mucous otitis media is found together with cholesteatoma in a greater number of cases than mere coincidence would allow. It is not exceptional to find a cholesteatoma in the tympanic cavity during the insertion of a ventilation tube or paracentesis for acute otitis.

Discovery of cholesteatoma during exploration of the tympanic cavity: When exploring the tympanic cavity in a case of conductive deafness, it is possible to find a cholesteatoma behind a tympanic membrane having a perfectly normal appearance. This is why, in a case of unilateral conductive deafness with a normal tympanic membrane, and no on-off effect on either side, radiological examination is desirable, comprising at least a Schüller's view; it may provide presumptive evidence, such as sclerotic mastoid, which makes it possible to question a diagnosis of otosclerosis and to turn rather towards the sequelae of inflammatory processes. There are, however, rare but not exceptional cases where diagnosis can only be reached by surgery.

Radiological Examination

The cholesteatoma develops within the bony cavity. Radiological examination is very useful as an aid to diagnosis in the difficult cases mentioned above. But, above all, it alone specifies the extent of the lesions.

Technique
Considerable progress has been made in radiological examination

of the petrous bones, both in the technical precision of the plates and in the choice of position.

Conventional Radiography. The strict insistence on the quality of the clinical examination must be matched by the quality of the radiological examination. From this point of view the use of the craniograph and of a 0.5-mm focus are indispensable. The main projections to be recommended are: (a) Schüller's projection: a lateral view which explores the squamous bone and assesses the pneumatization or eburnation of the mastoid; (b) Chausse III: an anteroposterior view which explores the attic-aditus-antrum area, and (c) Guillen's transorbital projection: an anteroposterior view, complementary to the preceding view, which explores the overall opacity of the chain, the supra- and retrotympanic spur, and the internal wall of the aditus.

Tomography. It is particularly in this field that technical possibilities have considerably developed. In chronological order, we have seen the arrival of linear scanning, circular scanning, hypocycloidal scanning, spiraled scanning, CGR Stratomatic, and Siemens Optiplanimat. The choice of projection: frontal plane, sagittal plane, parallel to the short axis of the temporal bone, and horizontal – Dulac VII (topography of the ossicular chain compared to the attic).

CT Scanning. High resolution CT scanning gives now better images than tomography. Obviously this list does not imply the necessity of using all the projections in every case. In the interests of medical economy it is better to proceed step by step rather than ask for a complete examination at the outset. A judicious and rational selection will make for a precise diagnosis, and it is advisable to consider the indications.

Indications
What, in concrete terms, can the otologist expect from a radiological exploration? In a general way, radiography can help him in (a) making the diagnosis; (b) judging the extent of the lesions, and (c) clarifying the indications for surgery and fixing the prognosis.

(a) *Making the diagnosis:* The assistance provided by radiology is extremely valuable in certain special cases described above in which it provides information that clinical examination cannot, e.g. otitis externa, narrowing of the meatus through congenital malformation or exostosis, or intact tympanic membrane cholesteatoma. It is perhaps useful to stress again the fact that diagnosis of cholesteatoma is made first and foremost by otoscopy. The otologist must not ask the radiologist to make up for a clinical inadequacy. It is not logical to have a conventional and tomographic examination carried out on an ear which has not first been examined through a microscope.

(b) *Judging the extent of the damage:* If a practised operator follows the matrix of the cholesteatoma step by step, he will discover the extent of the lesions much more precisely than he can from the information provided by radiology. Generally, he need rarely refer to this. Extension to the temporal bone poses a special problem. The usual seat of cholesteatoma is in the attic, the tympanic cavity, the antrum, and the tip of the mastoid. An extension way be observed towards the apex of the petrous bone (above, below, behind or within the labyrinth), the squamous temporal bone, the hypotympanum and the Eustachian tube. These are exceptional cases. Estimations of their frequency vary from 0.5 to 3%. Despite their rarity they are a constant concern. They call for a particular therapeutic attitude: middle fossa approach for extensions above the labyrinth, rerouting of the facial nerve for those below.

(c) *Clarifying the indications for surgery and fixing the prognosis:* Schüller's view, by showing the extent of eburnation or the degree of pneumatization of the mastoid and of the root of the zygoma, provides information which, depending on the clinical data, may assist the choice of technique. A sclerotic mastoid with complete destruction of the attic wall, which is generally accompanied by insufficiency of the Eustachian tube, gives rise, when using a closed technique, to difficult technical conditions, with instability of the reconstruction of the meatus and possible long-term deterioration of the results through the appearance of a retraction pocket. Conversely, using an open technique will be made easier by the reduced size of the mastoid cavity. A pneumatized mastoid, on the other hand, even if the attic wall is destroyed, calls rather for the use of a closed technique.

The case of a labyrinthine fistula: The discovery of a labyrinthine fistula may modify the indications for surgery and give a slightly different prognosis. It is advisable not to delay surgery. Here again, radiography is just one part of the whole picture. It may bring to light signs which announce the development of a fistula by showing erosion of the labyrinthine capsule: prefistular changes. It may provide objective evidence of a fistula, and particularly of its site: the lateral semicircular canal, more rarely the superior semicircular canal or promontory. It must nonetheless be interpreted with caution. Effacement phenomena caused by the proximity of a large, less dense, cavity may lead to the appearance of misleading pictures. Interviewing the patient and examining him clinically provides information which is equally, if not more, reliable.

To sum up, the usefulness of the radiological examination appears to be indisputable, but must be seen in perspective: (a) in diagnosing a cholesteatoma, radiology provides information, but rarely proof; (b) it may show too much by revealing a large cavity without being able to presume what it contains, and (c) it may show too little, since it is difficult, if not impossible, to objectivize small cholesteatomas which have not yet caused any erosion of the bone.

Comments

When the diagnosis is obvious, and surgery indicated, the contribution that radiology can make is limited. It is universally agreed that the more complex explorations should be reserved for special cases, where they play an essential part, and where clinical examination is inadequate. It is difficult to ignore the effect of the cost of the more sophisticated explorations, and they should be used advisedly to achieve greater efficiency.

A routine radiological examination as part of the preoperative examination of a cholesteatoma is called for when searching for an extension into the petrous bone. It is difficult to give an objective definition of a minimum examination, in which safety and economy are reconciled and which will provide for a major extension into the petrous bone: (a) extension into the petrous bone is rare (0.5–3%); (b) a normal radiological examination is only relatively reliable; (c) although the irradiation involved in such an exploration may be tolerable, its cost still deserves consideration; (d) surgical intervention, lastly, which reveals lesions step by step, may in exceptional cases make it possible to complete the diagnosis. It nonetheless puts the operator in a delicate psychological situation if it is necessary to change the direction of approach during the course of the operation, and because the prognosis is quite different.

The importance accorded to these different factors varies from author to author, and from country to country. Here, as an example, is the unequivocal position taken up by Smyth [22] in his recent treatise on chronic otitis media: 'In many otologic centers, mastoid X-rays are made in every case of chronic otitis. Although there is no denying the advantage of well-performed tomography as a means of detecting a coexisting acoustic schwannoma, I believe that routine «straight» X-ray studies constitute a waste of money and time, irradiate the patient unnecessarily, and do very little to assist the surgeon in determining the presence of a cholesteatoma or in indicating its dimensions. Furthermore, X-rays are positively dangerous if relied upon as a means of excluding the presence of cholesteatoma.'

Different sources adopt slightly differing attitudes. Some, in the absence of certain particular clinical elements, never ask for a routine radiological examination. Most, however, prefer to have a Schüller projection and some tomographic frontal views.

Bacteriological Findings

Many publications have been devoted to the bacterial flora of the discharge. The almost unanimous conclusion is that pyogenic bacteria are usually present, with a high frequency (nearly two-thirds of all cases) of pyocyanea and anaerobic strains. Medical treatment – suction under the microscope and local applications of wide-spectrum antibiotic, antifungal and antiseptic solutions – is an excellent preparation for surgical treatment. There are, however, otorrhoeas which are stubborn or so copious as to give rise to fears of infection with a particularly resistant germ. In such cases, the advantage of taking a sample for bacteriological analysis is that it can identify the bacteria in question and the antibiogram will indicate possible responsiveness or resistance to antibiotic treatment, at least in vitro, and guide the consultant in his choice of treatment.

For most modern surgeons, operating on an ear during a period of active suppuration or on a dry ear does not significantly change the surgical indications or even the protocol. For some, a reasonable attitude is to give the patient prior medical treatment in order to reduce infection, particularly of the skin of the meatus, and to improve functional recovery. This is particularly true when using tympano-ossicular homografts. There is an obvious risk, on the other hand, in delaying surgery indefinitely because of suppuration, since the infection is sustained by the presence of cholesteatomous lesions. Purulent otorrhoea, if chronic, must be seen as a sign of the extension of the cholesteatoma.

Examination of Hearing

The aim of the surgical treatment of cholesteatoma is the complete removal of the epidermic tissue and accompanying lesions, and the prevention of complications and recurrence. To these, modern surgery has added, as objectives of equal importance, the maintenance and even improvement of hearing. Concern for this aspect is first shown by the surgeon in the accurate assessment of the state of the patient's hearing, of the extent to which it can be recovered, and of his needs in social life. The first interview with the patient will give a general idea of how well his hearing corresponds to his social needs. It will of course be completed with a tuning-fork test, which will give a preliminary idea of the value of the cochlear reserve, if any. Some of us find it more reliable from a qualitative point of view, only ascribing a quantitative value to audiometry. The audiometric examination is limited in practice to a pure-tone examination in cases which pose no particular problem. In certain circumstances, vocal audiometry, speech discrimination tests or cochlear tests may be carried out. Rainville's test is indispensable in establishing bone conduction in cases of bilateral conductive deafness. It is important, when choosing the operative technique, to be as familiar with the functional and pathological state of the opposite ear as with that of the ear undergoing surgery.

ENT and General Examination of the Patient

Examination of Eustachian tube function: Many attempts have been made to assess the functional state of the Eustachian tube, which, beyond any doubt, plays a decisive role in the pathology of the middle ear: (a) Valsalva's and Politzer's techniques and (b) Eustachian manometry (Holmquist) which is only possible when there is an associated perforation.

To date, no method has been found to be completely reliable in predicting the recovery of the physiological function of the Eustachian tube. The obstruction may be caused directly by lesions known to be reversible or curable: mucous oedema, polyp, atelectatic tympanic membrane, or cholesteatoma. It is certain that permeability is not the only factor to be taken into consideration in the physiology of the middle ear. Other factors, such as gaseous exchange, ciliary or muscular physiology and immune reactions, must play a part which is still ill understood even less well known clinically, and even further from the sphere of our therapeutic acts. Examination of the opposite ear may provide, by analogy, valuable information.

State of the Nose and Throat

It is of the utmost importance to make a detailed examination of the state of the nose and throat, by questioning and examining the patient, in order to appreciate the background and to correct, where possible, obvious physiological disorders. A cleft palate or bifid uvula is prima facie evidence of permanent dysfunction of the Eustachian tube.

General Examination

The patient's general state of health should be assessed during a preoperative examination, by questioning the patient, by routine biological tests, and by any complementary examinations made necessary by the existence of any concomitant disorder. Aggravating factors (diabetes, old age, debility, 21-trisomy, Turner's syndrome, etc.) require special consideration and influence surgical indications and the choice of technique. An unruly child may require a general anesthetic for microscopic examination.

Complications

This chapter on the complications of cholesteatoma of the middle ear cannot be avoided, since even today between 20 and 25% of cases are involved. Quite frequently it is the appearance of the complication which first leads the patient to seek medical advice. At the risk of repeating ourselves to a certain extent, we shall consider here the more important pathogenic and clinical data, in the extent to which they can clarify the treatment to be applied.

Complications of cholesteatoma may either be infectious or take the form of a pseudo-tumour, whether the process has its seat within the temporal bone or whether it spreads further. They have become relatively less common since the introduction of antibiotics. They even appear to be less severe than was formerly the case. Ideas of treatment have evolved concurrently with theses changes.

When dealing with a cholesteatoma, a good otologist must be particularly careful. He must steer clear of both light-heartedness and overdramatization, and it is his duty to inform his patient as objectively as possible. Although complications may be less common than before, thanks to the progress made in ear surgery, it is still necessary to be careful.

Before antibiotics came into general use, the percentage of otogenic intracranial complications was 4% at the beginning of the century and 2.5% before the Second World War. In 1952, Jeanes put the percentage at 0.15%. Chronic otitis media is responsible for two-thirds of these complications and cholesteatoma is by far the biggest cause, particularly because of its ability to erode the bony structures unnoticed. The complications may therefore occur with lightning-like suddenness in a patient who is either neglectful or used to a more or less latent pathology of the ear.

General

A distinction should be made between two pathogenic mechanisms: (1) the growth of the cholesteatoma, which may go unnoticed, with only minimal inflammatory reaction, and develop into a pseudotumour, and (2) infection which is limited by the capsule over a long period prepares the way for the bacteria to spread continuously: if this matrix is burst by granulation tissue, the bacteria are immediately in a position where they can set to work, either directly or by following preformed pathways (the temporal bone is virtually 'honeycombed') when the vascular pathways have not made it possible for them to progress contiguously.

Other elements in a typical analysis are:

(1) The type of bacteria concerned and their sensitivity to antibiotics. Advances in the treatment of the infectious complications of chronic otitis media have been helped further by improved bacteriological knowledge, particularly in the part played by the gram-negative bacteria and above all in the improved identification of anaerobic bacteria.

(2) The individual response to the infection whose basic elements are extremely complex: tissue toxins, local enzyme response, and general metabolic problems which influence local behaviour.

(3) The drainage which is a relatively misleading criterion in clinical assessment. Although it is obvious that a mass of infected epithelial tissue or a polyp are effects of infection and favour the propagation of bacteria, it must not be thought that the marsupialization of a large mastoid cavity is a real protection. Cases of labyrinthine fistulae or facial paralysis are not exceptional, and we have even seen meningitis or cerebral abscesses on old operation cavities.

(4) Radiological examination, which is not an absolute criterion. Extremely cellular mastoids, with thin walls, are without doubt open to infection. A highly sclerotic mastoid, on the other hand, may be penetrated by a sheet of epidermic tissue which is not always easy to detect by radiography, even tomography. Bone erosion, by progressive enzymatic resorption, is actually more common than pyogenic osteitis in the vicinity of a cholesteatoma. In general the former precedes the latter. It will of course be much more rapid if the area around the matrix contains a large number of inflammatory elements and mobile cells. It is very difficult to lay down rules and predict how the bone will react to the invasion of epithelial tissue. It is in a state of constant change, and zones of reconstruction of bone tissue are found alongside

zones where the bone is becoming rarefied, sometimes giving macroscopic appearances reminiscent of osteoma.

(5) A certain number of otoscopic features which point more than others to the possibility of complications: deep-seated lesions of the attic, for example, persistent suppuration, recurrent polyps or stubbornly fetid otorrhoea.

The complications of cholesteatoma are well known, and we shall dwell only on those points which are controversial. In the context of the modern approach to cholesteatoma, it would seem to be more important to clarify those ideas which must be constantly borne in mind. Surgery is indicated nowadays at an increasingly earlier stage. This is justified but it is also important to avoid this 'interventionism' becoming itself a cause of complications.

Premonitory Symptoms of Complications

The development of public health measures covering the whole of the population has not had the corollary effect of improving hygiene in certain patients or eliminating the neglect shown by others suffering from chronic otitis media. Since effective prevention can only be achieved through education, it is unfortunately probable that this state of affairs will remain with us for a long time, even in the so-called developed countries. In chronic otitis media, the patient's attitude to hygiene is a very important element, which is in fact unrelated to his intellectual or economic status, being rather a true reflection of his ability to understand the necessity for discipline. An experienced otologist will only propose sophisticated surgery to a patient whom he deems to be sufficiently 'reliable'.

Signs Which Alert

When it accompanies a polypoid reaction, bleeding will often alarm the patient. Otalgia is a symptom of a local outbreak of infection – otitis externa, rekindling of inflammation or failure of drainage. The rekindled inflammation, whether or not it is accompanied by any recrudescence of the otorrhoea, whether it is secondary to an infection of the nose and throat or to contamination from outside, is always a sign of the progression of granulation tissue around the matrix, and therefore of a speeding-up of the process of bone resorption. Favoured by such an occurrence, the matrix itself may be burst, favouring dispersal of the bacteria. Persistence of a fetid discharge is generally a sign of extension of the cholesteatoma, and it must be emphasized that radiography always underestimates the importance of the lesions.

Signs Which Warn

The threat may be more or less definite, but the surgeon must always be on the lookout, particularly as the vast majority are found during routine general examinations, and routine tends to dull the clinical senses. It is rather remarkable (a) that most life-threatening intracranial complications occur in patients who have rarely seen an otologist and are often admitted to neurosurgery or infectious diseases wards once the complication has occurred, and (b) that the clinical forms of certain life-threatening complications, especially abscesses, may be atypical – a relative deterioration of the general state of health, or an unexplained loss of weight may be indicators.

Particular attention will be given to: (a) Headache – this is a non-specific symptom, but it must always be carefully investigated in any patient suffering from chronic otitis media, even if it occurs in isolation with no other accompanying signs. It must be distinguished from otalgia: it is often in the temporal or occipitomastoid region. It is more dragging than actually painful: there is a feeling of deep-seated, ill-defined heaviness. (b) Changing in behaviour, such as irritability or, on the contrary, asthenia and sleepiness. These must be looked for systematically. (c) Fever – even if only moderate, this is a potential danger sign.

When these warning signs occur in isolation, in no particular general or neurological context, it is advisable to proceed to special deep investigations, bearing in mind: (a) that the EEG can only localize lesions above the tentorium; (b) that gamma scanning is very useful in diagnosing and localizing abscesses; (c) that CT scanning, which is becoming more and more easily available, has revolutionized possibilities of diagnosis by its precision and speed, and (d) that arteriography is still valuable when there is no CT scanner available.

Intratemporal Complications

This type of complication in nowadays the most common, and may be classified, from a clinical point of view, into two groups:

Complications Connected with Extension of the Cholesteatoma

These complications cause disorders of function. Such complications generally occur at the site of previous lesions, as a result of the exposure of the facial nerve within the petrous bone or of erosion of the labyrinthine capsule. Facial paralysis (FP) or vertigo may occur suddenly with no modification of the clinical picture – otorrhoea is minimal or absent, and there are no headaches or signs of failure of drainage.

FP occurred in 0.5% of cases of acute otitis, and 1.7% of cases of chronic otitis media before the advent of antibiotics. In Forni's [79] thesis, there is a percentage of 1.75% over 400 cases. 80% of cases of otogenic FP nowadays are linked to the presence of a cholesteatoma. It may be considered that they are favoured by anatomical dehiscence of the facial nerve canal (50% of petrous bones) but in most cases the cholesteatoma itself is the eroding agent. In the absence of any serious infectious phenomenon, the tolerance of the nerve trunk is remarkable.

Electrical tests of facial nerve function do not always give the same picture of induction block, since FP may occur without any great deterioration in the wall of the bony canal, by venous congestion and oedema. When the canal is open, for the same degree of motor dysfunction, the actual lesions may vary a great deal: the nerve may just as easily be whitish and atonic as red and oedematous. It is rare for the perineurium to be destroyed, and for inflammatory granulomas to pass inside and to disrupt the nerve fibres. In some cases, examination of the state of the perineurium during surgery is not easy, and requires great care and caution. Exploration of the canal of the facial nerve must be complete and will generally be guided by the lesions. It must be noted:

(1) That the bony canal must be opened on both sides of the lesion in order to reach the zone where the perineurium is healthy.

(2) That some of us are of the opinion that an intact or only slightly modified perineurium should not be incised. Why should the facial nerve be an exception when the perineurium is never opened in surgery of the peripheral nerves? In the circumstances with which we are concerned here, opening the perineurium brings with it a high risk of opening the nerve trunk to invasion by inflammatory cells.

(3) That a granuloma which disrupts the perineurium must be dissected. Although the facial nerve may literally be broken into strands,

especially in the first portion, we have never (apart from cases of ia-trogenic problems) met with a break in the nerve trunk. We shall not tackle the question of the repair of the facial nerve here, as it is a special problem.

(4) That the absence of important lesions of the perineurium is quite compatible with a closed technique when the other anatomical conditions are favourable.

(5) That a fistula of the lateral canal is sometimes also present and that, in these conditions, an open technique is the wisest solution.

(6) That the presence of paralysis does not in itself determine the choice of technique which is dependent, essentially, on the accompanying lesions.

In any event, the recent appearance of facial paralysis during the development of a cholesteatoma constitutes an urgent indication for surgery. It will nonetheless be remembered: (a) that electroneurography and computerized electromyography are desirable, since other investigations are of little value at this stage; (b) that bacteriological samples should be taken systematically and followed by an antibiogram, and (c) that rarer diagnoses, sometimes relying on intraoperative, histological examination such as tuberculosis or cancer, must never be discounted.

A labyrinthine fistula (LF) is almost always situated in the lateral semicircular canal. The proportion of LF found elsewhere is less than 10% – in decreasing order of frequency and increasing order of seriousness, they may be found in the superior canal, posterior canal, promontory, oval window or the anterior cochlea.

The fistula makes its appearance in a stealthy manner, and the matrix of the cholesteatoma erodes the labyrinthine capsule so slowly that it serves at the same time as a cover and as a temporary protection from possible infection. In such circumstances the patient himself is often the first to trigger off the fistula sign by applying fortuitous pressure to the tragus or while cleaning the meatus. In 80% of cases, even when the test for LF is negative, questioning the patient will reveal that he suffers from vertigo and slight loss of balance.

It is indeed often difficult to apply the fistula test, or it may vary from one day to the next. Different authors give positive results between 40 and 60% of cases of LF. It must be remembered:

(1) That LF is even today a complication in about 10% of cholesteatomas. This is ample justification for routinely testing for LF when-

ever a cholesteatoma sufferer seeks medical advice. McCabe [144] has applied it successfully 32 times out of 35 cases of fistula using technical refinements including electronystagmography.

(2) That the test for LF can only be applied with a positive result before surgery in 50% of cases on average. The absence of a positive response does not thus necessarily imply the absence of a fistula. Once in every 20 operations, therefore, the surgeon has a statistical chance of discovering a 'surprise fistula'. This fact means that particular care must be taken when operating in 'high risk' zones, in order to avoid being taken by surprise [81]. Theoretically, of course, a tomographical examination may be carried out on any cholesteatoma, but in practice, caught as we are between the need to limit the costs and the requirements of that medical perfectionism with which we are increasingly reproached today, a certain number of cholesteatomas are operated on with only a Schüller's projection. It must also be emphasized that tomography, even when of excellent quality, may conceal some details. One of the present authors was recently operating on a cholesteatoma with a positive fistula test; tomography showed a highly suspect zone in the superior semicircular canal, while the convexity of the lateral semicircular canal appeared to be intact. In the course of the operation it was found that the fistula was actually situated over the ampulla of the lateral semicircular canal.

At the first stage of its development, a LF is not accompanied by any notable vestibular disturbance, and the main benefit of the ENG recording is to bring out Lucae's sign, if it is present. There is of course no question of ignoring the danger involved. There can be no doubt of the indication for surgery when a LF is present. The presence of even the slightest inflammatory reaction, causing the liberation of toxic substances, and the presence of adjacent infected lesions may destabilize the situation from one moment to the next and lead to labyrinthine failure. Although Neely [151] speaks of chronic labyrinthitis, we prefer to keep the classical term of 'paralabyrinthitis'. This appears to us to be an important distinction, particularly as experience has shown us that inner ear function may be perfectly preserved after the operation. Although the presence of a fistula may potentially pose a serious threat, it does not justify the defeatist attitude of radical surgery, but rather means that the otologist must be more careful and watchful [238]. Statistics provided by one of the present authors [251], dealing with 100 cases of fistula of the lateral semicircular canal, show (a) that the opposite ear is affected in 70% of cases, and that in 50% of these the condition gives cause for concern, since a cholesteatoma is also present; (b) it sometimes happens that the opposite ear is totally deaf, or so severely affected that we are obliged to operate on the patient's only functional ear, and (c) that the cochlear reserve of the ear affected by the fistula determines the degree to which preservation of hearing may be expected. In his statistics, one of the present authors has noticed that such ears are deaf in 22% of cases, and that 27% of them have a level of bone conduction which is above 30 dB. In his series, Ritter [176] notes 30% of cases of deafness.

It is nonetheless true that, five times out of ten, the cochlear reserve is suffcient to justify a concerted approach aimed at preserving the hearing without minimizing the difficulties of the problem. It is true that large series are rare in the literature on the subject, and that opinions differ on the following four questions: (1) Should the matrix be preserved to protect the fistula? (2) Should we rather take a 'calculated risk', with all the necessary technical precautions, and routinely remove the epithelium from the fistula, at the risk of causing damage to the inner ear? (3) What, depending on the solution adopted, is the long-term future of the cochlear reserve? (4) What, when a fistula is present, are the limitations of the open and closed techniques, respectively?

The reader must refer to the chapter on surgical techniques but (and although we may be repeating ourselves here) the course of action when a LF (still the commonest complication of cholesteatoma) is present requires particular consideration in view of what is currently possible from a technical point of view.

In a study of 50 cases, Ritter [176] advises that the matrix should not be removed. Palva et al. [158], Gacek [83], and Abramson et al. [7] recommend complete removal of the cholesteatoma when a fistula is present, emphasizing that the real problem for the future, which must not be shirked, is to cure the chronic otitis media. One of the present authors has found that 12% of fistulae appear in old mastoidectomy cavities and stresses that the thinness of the dystrophic epithelium is not a sufficient long-term guarantee. He therefore suggests complete removal, except when dealing with the only hearing ear. Dissection of the matrix is carried out at the first stage of open-technique surgery or during the revision stage in closed-technique surgery. It must be noted that dissection of the matrix at the second stage (whether in open- or closed-technique surgery) may present unsuspected problems, e.g., (a) difficulty in finding a plane of cleavage; (b) the possibility of finding osteomatous reactions on the edges which may make removal of the matrix hazardous; (c) occasionally, extension of the fistula, and (d) finally, when using a closed technique, some authors have reported, at the second stage, the disappearance (verified by histological examination) of all traces of epithelium from the fistula. Such accounts are, in fact, anecdotal.

In 1978, Sheehy [206] reported his dual experience – systematic removal of the matrix from 1967 to 1973, then preservation. He reviewed 97 cases in the hope of finding an answer to this problem, and observed that, in his operations, the percentage of deafness was the same whichever method was used. He wrote: '...to state with assurance that one or other method of operative management is preferable: we cannot.'

In 1980, Smyth [219] took up the discussion once more, favouring preservation of the matrix: (a) using closed-technique surgery wherever possible, with removal of the matrix during revision: 2 cases of deafness and one deterioration out of 22 cases, and (b) using an open technique particularly when operating on the only hearing ear, and without attempting to reconstruct the tympanum or ossicular chain (no modification of bone conduction in any one of 25 cases).

We consider that the discussion is not closed, and that different types of cases should be treated differently. Out of a series of over 100 cases reported in 1974, involving systematic removal of the matrix, one of the present authors [251] observed that bone conduction was lowered by more than 20 dB in 15%, and was completely preserved in 80%. Subsequent experience, benefiting from the lessons learned from this series, has only served to confirm the soundness of his approach. We may consider:

(1) That the matrix may be dissected with the minimum of risk if strict technical rules are observed (bloodless fields, no suction in the vicinity of the window, and dissection of the matrix at the very last moment of the operation). From a functional point of view, results are often excellent, and in some cases bone conduction is improved. The fistula often closes subsequently.

(2) That preservation of the matrix most often provides a false sense of security in the short term, and an uncertain long-term future. This method is justified when operating on the only hearing ear, when

obvious and active infection is present, and if the fistula spread beyond the lateral semicircular canal, or has its seat elsewhere. When the fistula spreads beyond the limits of the lateral semicircular canal, Sheely [206] notes deafness in 5 out of 9 cases.

(3) That routine dissection of the fistula is only justifiable when the surgeon is particularly experienced, and that, finally, the labyrinth will be better protected by a graft of connective tissue (perichondrium rather than fascia in our opinion) than by a matrix whose future is uncertain.

Infectious Complications

Since the chronicity of the suppuration is part of the clinical picture, we shall only consider here those acute infectious complications which, within a few hours or a few days, can completely change the clinical picture and prognosis of a chronic otorrhoea which may have appeared relatively mild, or even have been completely ignored. We shall not take into account either the progressive sensorineural losses which take place over a period of years and cover the entire inflammatory pathology of the middle ear apart from cholesteatoma, or the problematical arachnoiditis of the cerebellopontine angle.

Conditions Affecting the Labyrinth

Acute Labyrinthitis. This is without doubt the complication which is most feared from a functional point of view. It may occur at any point during the development of a LF and represents the bursting of the matrix of the cholesteatoma – it is immediately purulent and presents a gloomy prognosis for the hearing.

In most cases, the spread of infection in the labyrinth is contiguous through the windows, or along vascular pathways. Changes in the perilymph are first biological, then cytological. A distinction is normally made between: (a) The stage of serous (or toxic) labyrinthitis which might in theory be reabsorbed with no sequelae. In fact it favours a process of slowly progressing fibrosis, and its more attenuated form probably explains the cochlear regression which, slight though it may be, is so often observed in clinical examination, independent of and prior to any surgical act. Tympanoplasty may very well accompany the removal of the lesions. (b) The stage of acute suppurative labyrinthitis which develops quickly as soon as the bacteria themselves reach the cavities of the labyrinth, to end, in the complete form, in necrosis of the membranous labyrinth. Two bacteria are particularly dangerous because of their ability to penetrate the meninges – *Pneumococcus* and *Haemophilus influenzae*. The infection spreads along the vestibular nerves or through the basal extremity of the scala tympani and the modiolus.

Antibiotics cannot preserve function at the stage of suppurative labyrinthitis, but they have led to a situation where it is very rare to encounter meningitis as a consequence of a labyrinthitis whose origin lies in a condition affecting the middle ear. When it is a complication of the development of a cholesteatoma, labyrinthitis is generally purulent, in a setting of acute vestibular symptoms with fever. It is generally possible to carry out an audiogram, with the patient in his bed if necessary, to complete the examination. When such a picture is present, there is a definite indication for surgery, but this must not be precipitate. First of all, any other associated complication, for which the labyrinthitis may well serve as starting-point, must be eliminated – especially meningitis or brain abscess. Intravenous broad-spectrum antibiotic therapy is immediately put into operation, ensuring a respite of at least 24 h in all cases. From a surgical point of view, a radical mastoidectomy is compulsory. Formal labyrinthectomy is no longer in vogue nowadays unless in following the lesion the surgeon opens the labyrinth as part of his procedure.

Chronic labyrinthitis develops slowly: (a) Either as a sequela of a serous labyrinthitis whose degree may vary greatly depending on whether the process is confined to the perilymph or involves the organ of Corti. This is affected first at the basal turn with damage to the outer hair cells which are most vulnerable. The clinical and audiometric situation may appear stable over a long period, but vestibular tests will often show persistent signs of irritation with no tendency to compensation. As the years go by, there is a gradual deterioration of cochlear function, which may sometimes suddenly accelerate for no apparent reason. (b) Or in the context of a LF. Loss of substance from the bony capsule makes contact and invasion by connective tissue easier. Bacteria may invade at any moment, allowing the condition to develop into suppurative labyrinthitis. The expression 'walled-off labyrinthitis' ('labyrinthite cloisonnée' in French) has been used to describe this type of sudden, unexpected development.

Sclerosis of the Labyrinth. This is defined as an active stage following labyrinthitis. Its intensity depends on the severity with which the labyrinth has been affected. Fibrosis reinforces the granulation tissue in the bony cavities. It is always extensive in the basal region. When the lesion has been severe, there is metaplasia into bone and it is possible to speak of 'labyrinthitis ossificans'.

From the moment the functions of the cochlea and vestibule disappear, the otologist has no clinical evidence which can allow him to assess the extent of the process. One of the present authors has observed a patient with a facial paralysis whose history had started 13 years previously with a transient hemispasm. A neurologist advised the patient to consult an otologist, but she neglected to take this step. Seven years later she presented severe symptoms of Ménière's disease for 8 days. No otological examination was carried out. Two years after this incident an otologist observed deafness, but was content with cleaning the meatus. Three years later the appearance of the FP made the patient decide to undergo surgery, during which it was observed that there was complete destruction of the lateral and posterior semicircular canals.

Acute Mastoiditis. This is rare as a complication of the development of a cholesteatoma. In adults, especially when the cholesteatoma sac has the typical form of a pseudo-tumour, there may be extension into the postaural sulcus, or collapse of the posterosuperior wall of the meatus. This is not acute mastoiditis, but a pseudo-tumour. In children, acute mastoiditis extending subcutaneously has itself become rare. The proportion of such cases which reveal latent and even massive cholesteatomas has thus assumed greater significance. In any event, there is a definite indication for surgery. The surgeon must bear in mind that 'one lesion may conceal another'. He must not be content with a routine mastoidectomy and should explore the permeability of the interatticotympanic diaphragm, check Schrapnell's membrane and explore the posterior part of the tympanic cavity.

Chronic mastoiditis accompanies, in varying degrees, any cholesteatoma which has reached and blocked the aditus area. Human pathology reproduces Beaumont's [17] experiments perfectly. In practice, all the different stages in the reaction of the mucosa and the bone may be found, namely coalescent mastoiditis, cholesterol granuloma, and osteogenic reaction.

Temporal Bone Cholesteatomas

Certain cholesteatomas, generally in the attic, grow slowly and progressively like a pseudo-tumour. The starts and stops in epithelial growth may be explained by the relative strength of the otic capsule, by the heterogeneity of the structures, especially in highly pneumatized mastoids, and as a result of individual differences in bone metabolism. They may spread unsuspected beyond the limits of the temporal bone and become apparent: (a) by extension subcutaneously as we have just seen – external mastoid cortex, posterior wall of the meatus, very rarely the foot of the squamous bone, and exceptionally the root of the zygoma; (b) by upwards and backwards extension following the shape of the posterior part of the labyrinth to appear in the suprapetrous region, eroding the roof of the antrum or the aditus, to erode the inside of the internal auditory meatus (double pouch shape); (c) by extension forwards and above the cochlea towards the geniculate ganglion. In some cases, the posterior part of the labyrinth is decapitated at the semicircular canals, and the internal auditory meatus is directly penetrated, while, paradoxically, the facial nerve may resist for quite some time, although it may be exposed to a large extent. These forms may be revealed by symptoms which falsely suggest Ménière's disease, deafness, atypical facial pains, or a facial hemispasm. In some cases, conductive deafness observed in association with irregular facial spasms will point to the diagnosis. Nager [150] points out that repeated aseptic meningeal reactions may be associated; (d) by extension downwards and forwards into the hypotympanic region with exposure of the superior bulb of the internal jugular vein, of the carotid, and possible extension into the peritubal cells.

If there are no localizing signs, the extension of the cholesteatoma around the petrous bone can only be diagnosed. (a) By frontal tomography, particularly for extensions above the labyrinth. The radiological appearance is fairly characteristic: the bone destruction has regular contours which are sometimes slightly sclerotic, especially in less pneumatized mastoids. (b) Sometimes, it is only through surgical exploration that the diagnosis can be made, when the radiological examination has been insufficient and when, in the absence of clinical signs, only a conventional Schuller's projection has been used in order to limit costs.

When, even with a reasonable radiological examination, the epithelial invasion is in the form of a 'sheet', the radiological image is sometimes difficult to analyze: this is as true when, with a sclerotic or eburnated mastoid, epithelial tissue penetrates between two blocks of sclerotic bone, as it is when, with a highly pneumatized mastoid, the superimposition of layers of varying densities makes detailed analysis difficult. One must be wary of labyrinthine capsules which appear relatively sclerotic.

Finally, it must be remembered that the existence of an unstable mastoidectomy cavity must not be allowed to divert attention from the possibility that the cholesteatoma has extended to the petrous bone. If there is the slightest doubt, only tomography can bring this out. The same is theoretically true when imperfectly executed closed-technique surgery has not been followed by a systematically planned second-look operation.

Signs of localization appear relatively late, and the surgeon is always struck by the size of the extension compared to the paucity of the symptoms: (a) the otoscopic changes are sometimes very slight; (b) often the only signs are slight facial myoclonus and a few pains in the trigeminal or retro-orbital area; (c) major involvement of the cochlea, and indeed deafness, should arouse suspicion; (d) even when there are no labyrinthine, cochlear or vestibular signs, tomography or surgery may sometimes reveal decapitation of the semicircular canals or a cochlear fistula; (e) according to Fisch [71], a severe lesion of the facial nerve usually corresponds with a lesion of its intralabyrinthine part, which may be divided into strands; nerve graft with rerouting is justified in such cases.

These otoneurosurgical forms of cholesteatoma of the middle ear are almost always the result of attic lesions. There is in fact no correlation between the otoscopic appearance and the degree of inward extension of the cholesteatoma. One of the present authors recently observed a case which is instructive in this context: a 65-year-old man suffered from chronic suppuration until the age of 25. A regular soldier, he noticed that each time he experienced a detonation in a closed space (firing range), he suffered a sudden, brief loss of balance (a true sign of LF), then this went away although hearing in this ear disappeared progressively. The patient therefore only sought medical advice 30 years later, as he was then suffering from facial paralysis, when he had a large, double pouch-shaped cholesteatoma.

In some cases, differential diagnosis is difficult in cases of congenital cholesteatomas of the petrous bone with secondary extension to the middle ear. Cody [47] estimates that 98% of cases of cholesteatoma of the petrous bone originate in the middle ear. The same view is held by Sterkers and Sterkers [231]. In fact, when there is no infection, they pose the same problems as primary cholesteatomas of the petrous bone, as we shall see. The approach will be determined by the type of extension, the infection, and the possibility of dissecting the matrix.

Type of Extension

(1) Extension above and behind the labyrinth is by far the most common type, sometimes accompanied by lesions within the labyrinth. Whatever the state of hearing may be, the translabyrinthine approach is to be avoided unless it is necessary in order to follow the lesions. The essential principle in dissecting the cholesteatoma is always to approach and even go beyond its limits, especially inwards [232].

In the view of Fisch [71] the state of hearing is a criterion in the choice of the approach. If the inner ear is fully functional, he prefers the middle fossa approach combined with an open-technique tympanoplasty ('transmastoid modified radical operation') to drain and then keep under observation. When there is a deafness, this author suggests a posterior translabyrinthine approach, sacrificing the posterior wall of the meatus and maintaining the tympanic membrane.

In the view of the present authors, whatever the state of the hearing may be, and as long as the removal of the cholesteatoma is complete, preference should be given to the closed technique as for a congenital cholesteatoma. Unless it is forced upon the surgeon by the anatomical conditions, the creation of a large cavity can only have disadvantageous results, in particular that of secondary infection. The growth of any residue from the matrix will be much slower if it is closed in than if it is in indirect contact with the exterior. As early as 1949, Olivecrona followed up 6 cases of cholesteatoma after partial removal of the matrix, without any recurrence after 10 years. There is no doubt that such an attitude is arguable. It must be applied intelligently, but with tomography and the latest generation of CT scanners at our disposal, we think that it constitutes the ideal to aim for, since long-term observation is becoming possible.

As soon as the superior semicircular canal is affected, the postaural approach is insufficient. It is necessary to start by a middle fossa approach. A second principle, stressed by Sterkers, is to identify the facial nerve both above and below the cholesteatoma.

(2) Anterosuperior extension towards the geniculate ganglion: middle fossa approach whatever the state of the hearing.

(3) Extension beneath the labyrinth (or cochlea) are luckily rare but their treatment is difficult. The need for complete eradication makes it necessary to use a infratemporal approach with rerouting of the VII, using the technique suggested by Fisch [73].

The problem posed by infection is more theoretical than real. Gacek [84] and Fisch [71] suggest for drainage, even for primary cholesteatomas of the petrous bone. The attitude to be adopted will be decided in the light of the circumstances of each particular case. Cholesteatomas extending inside the petrous bone are rarely deeply infected and generally take a tumour-like form. Insofar as is possible, they must be treated with a closed technique, which is possible in the majority of cases by using a double approach – middle fossa and transmastoid – with repair of the tegmen. Some, however, prefer to sacrifice the posterior canal wall routinely. Where there is extension within or beneath the labyrinth requiring Fisch's technique, suppression of the external auditory meatus and canal is a perfectly justifiable attitude in the circumstances (Rambo's 'obliteration').

Adhesion of the Matrix

It is rare to find that the matrix cannot be totally dissected. There is certain to be difficulty with the wall of the lateral sinus and the meninges. When the surface is small, resection with repair of the meninges may be envisaged. The decision to marsupialize via a radical mastoidectomy is only to be taken with regret, as follow-up and inspection are done for appearance sake rather than with true effect. Deep-seated invasion may continue unobserved, beyond the view of the speculum.

Infectious Intracranial Complications

We have already seen that the otologist must always be concerned with signs which are premonitory of complications and with their analysis: an unexplained deterioration of general health, changes in behaviour, fever even when only moderate, and especially persistent and dragging headaches. In practice, it must always be stressed today: (a) that intratemporal complications (FP and LF) require surgery and that they are now no longer the starting-point of other complications by contiguous extension, and (b) that the ENT area is the most common site of etiology of brain abscesses and secondary meningitis, without any strict correlation with the local process. Their spread is most often contiguous (by vascular pathways), favoured by the nature of the bacteria (anaerobic bacteria which are better studied today by bacteriology laboratories).

The ENT surgeon should routinely seek the collaboration of the neurologist and/or the neurosurgeon in diagnosing the nature and localization of the complication. Nevertheless, it is regrettable that even today a very careful ENT examination is not carried out routinely on every patient suffering from meningitis or intracerebral suppuration. One of the present authors has had a patient, albeit an awkward one, who presented with a productive cholesteatoma of the attic 2 years after the removal of an encapsulated temporal abscess! The general attitude to be adopted when an infectious intracranial complication is present has varied from time and time and from school to school. It should be decided in consultation with the neurosurgery and clinical bacteriology departments. The order of treatment depends primarily on the life expectancy and often the complication will be the first to be treated. Some authors always give priority to the otological area. In the view of others it must follow as soon as possible, and as soon as the patient's state of health allows it, after the treatment of the complication.

We shall therefore confine ourselves here, with an apology for its somewhat didactic nature, to a mere summary: The *extradural abscess* is a suppurative collection of limited volume, situated between the bone and the dura mater, generally around the tegmen and the lateral sinus, and often in direct communication with the infected mastoid cells. Less commonly the surgeon may note a granulomatous appearance of the dural surface. It is often asymptomatic. Symptoms are often limited to a persistent heaviness of the ear, with radiation to the temporal, retro-orbital or occipital regions. An ill-defined feeling of general discomfort or an intermittent, unobtrusive febrile state should be looked for.

In children, the symptoms are more numerous: a certain degree of lassitude may be observed, with a meningeal syndrome. The differential diagnosis should be made with an intracerebral abscess. This is very often a case where discovery is made during surgery. The open technique is required, and it is possible to preserve the tympanic cavity, depending on the lesions. The sole problem is the attitude to be adopted toward the loss of bone substance which, even if it is relatively limited, may favour a subsequent prolapse of the meninges. When there are limited lesions, we are of the opinion that, with the aid of elective antibiotic treatment, repair may be carried out immediately, with cartilage from the concha, for example.

A *subdural abscess* is rare. This is the accumulation of pus between the dura mater and the arachnoid. Differential diagnosis may be difficult with a diffuse meningitis, but the presence of certain signs of neurological localization, associated with an aseptic, cellular and protein reaction of the cerebrospinal fluid, may serve to direct the search in the right direction. The CT scanner and the arteriogram results are generally positive. Antibiotic treatment and neurosurgical drainage are required. The otological operation is carried out once the complication is under control or if the patient does not respond to treatment.

Thrombophlebitis of the lateral sinus generally coexists with an extradural abscess in the vicinity. It is a localized inflammation of the vein wall which may be followed by thrombosis of the wall, then complete blockage of the lateral sinus. The thrombus may then form an abscess or disintegrate into emboli. This type of complication has become very rare nowadays and is above all connected with acute otitis. Fever, of the septicaemic type, is the most suggestive element in the diagnosis, which is verified at the venous stage of carotid arteriography. A radical operation is required, with complete cleaning of the infected thrombus. Antibiotic treatment makes it possible to avoid operating on a partial thrombosis when the appearance of the vein wall is satisfactory. Ligature of the internal jugular vein is carried out if there have been embolic problems.

Diffuse meningitis develops with a varying degree of rapidity, and may sometimes be violent. The three classical stages help guide the therapeutic approach with reference to a parallel study of the clinical picture and the state of the CSF:

(a) Serous meningeal reaction: the CSF is clear, but its pressure has increased. The patient presents a moderate meningeal syndrome, with no vomiting or signs of localization.

(b) Aseptic meningitis: the pressure of the CSF, which is sometimes cloudy or amber-coloured, is raised. The number of cells and proteins is considerably increased, with a reduction of chlorides. No bacteria are present, or, at least the bacteria are not always identified by the laboratory. The meningeal syndrome is clear-cut: violent headaches, drowsiness, photophobia and vomiting.

(c) Suppurative meningitis: the CSF is definitely cloudy, with increases in the numbers of cells and proteins, while the chloride and glucose contents are lowered. Above all, bacteria are found to be present on direct examination. Clinically, the patient has no reflexes and is often comatose. Immediate surgery is only justified at the stage of serous meningeal reaction, and possibly at the stage of aseptic cellular reaction, provided that it is carried out during the first few days when the patient can easily withstand the operation.

(d) Systematic search for associated complications: whatever the stage of development of the meningeal involvement, it must be remembered that other infectious complications may also be present, especially in older children and adults. The relative frequency of such multiple complications should mean that a systematic search is made for them. A meningitis may conceal the development of an abscess.

With this in mind, it is important to determine by which route the infection is spreading: this is of practical use and not merely academic interest. The sudden occurence of severe deafness with nystagmus, vertigo and vomiting tends to suggest that it is spreading by the preformed pathways of the vestibular cavities. Tomography of the petrous bone may give cause to suspect that infection is spreading directly, when there is a loss of substance from the tegmen. When both cochlea and vestibule are functioning properly, either direct extension or a retrograde thrombophlebitis may be suspected. These distinctions, by giving a better idea of the relationship between the otological seat and the involvement of the meninges, make it easier to decide on the treatment indicated – priority will be given to medical treatment if the spread of the infection is vascular, otherwise surgery, which should not be delayed too long provided that the patient's general state of health will withstand it, will be preferred. It should be noted that in cases of bilateral chronic otitis media, it is often difficult to determine which side is responsible for the infection. Unless there is an incontrovertible relationship, medical treatment of the complication is the first priority. It is preferable to cure the meningitis medically when cochlear function is intact and when the anatomical condition of the middle ear is not too disastrous. Surgery, with the aim of saving, and even improving, function, may be envisaged thereafter – an open technique will of course be used.

Cerebral or cerebellar abscess: Suppuration of the parenchyma of the temporal lobe or of the cerebellum may present appearances during the course of its development. The seat of the necrosis appears with varying degrees of rapidity, and, since it is always surrounded by an ill-defined zone of encephalitis, the tendency to encapsulation is slight. There may be multiple abscesses and there is a constant danger of rupture within the ventricular system. Otogenic central or cerebellar abscesses are rare and occur particularly during the second and third decades of life. Even today, the mortality rate is still 20% in most sets of statistics.

Direct extension with loss of substance from the tegmen is the most common mechanism but, since the dura mater is highly resistant, an extradural abscess, which often precedes the lesion in the parenchyma, will spread through a retrograde thrombophlebitis. Four stages of development are usually distinguished: (1) the invasion stage of initial encephalitis; (2) the stage of localization of the latent abscess; (3) the gathering, or manifest abscess, stage, and (4) the terminal rupture stage. At the first two stages, diagnosis may be easy, and the signs which alert and which warn (see above) must be analyzed. These signs may last for several weeks, after which the situation may take a dramatic turn. It will be remembered that CT scanning has become the key to diagnosis, but that it may show normal results in the initial stages, as indeed may arteriography. The EEG therefore is still valuable as a pointer in 75% of cases from the beginning. Treatment will be discussed with and carried out by the neurosurgeon, bearing in mind both the rise in intracranial pressure and the infection. In exceptional cases a surgical approach from below may be used to follow the lesions.

Current trends regarding intracranial suppuration: Fisch [73] estimates their frequency currently at 1.22% (out of 1,907 cases of chronic otitis media over a period of 20 years), while Georges et al. [89] stress the fact that ENT is the most common origin of brain abscesses (40.6%). Fisch emphasizes that 26% of his patients (6 out of 23) had already undergone ear surgery in a period of between 8 months and 5 years before the occurrence of the complication. In all these cases an open technique was used, which demonstrates clearly that a radical mastoidectomy is no guarantee against intracranial complications if the technique is inadequate, or if there is either a supravestibular or an infracochlear extension. In Fisch's view, with which the present authors entirely agree, a radical mastoidectomy requires as much anatomical knowledge and technical skill as does a closed technique. It may be thought surprising that infectious complications are not found as a result of closed-technique surgery, but Fisch's impression is confirmed by the recent work of Vaneecloo et al. [246], who have found a previous history of open-technique surgery in 5 out of 25 cases of otogenous brain abscesses (20%) [693].

Fisch goes as far as to write: 'If a closed cavity is modeled as an open one with the only exception of the preserved thin posterosuperior canal wall, the possible residual or recurrent cholesteatoma will not grow in depth, but rather break outwards through either the retroauricular skin or the external auditory canal.' This statement is no doubt somewhat categorical – at a time when the second-look operation was not in routine use, one of the present authors observed a double pouch-shaped supralabyrinthine cholesteatoma with no outward clinical appearance which was revealed by a fistula in the superior semicircular canal. It is nonetheless possible to maintain, without wishing to put forward a paradox, that, provided that the surgeon is competent and the patient will submit to regular follow-up, a buried fragment of matrix is no more dangerous than a marsupialized and infected cholesteatoma. With the benefit of hindsight we can see that the arguments against closed-technique surgery are more dogmatic than real. In fact, in the view of the present authors, there is nothing worse than improperly carried our open-technique surgery: this observation is, however, confined here to the particular case of complications affecting life expectancy.

In the preceding paragraphs we have given a somewhat didactic summary. In actual fact, CT scanning and improved bacteriological analyses identifying anaerobic bacteria have changed the practical approach. Many schools of neurosurgery gave preference to excision until 1978. Since then, Georges et al. [89] have stressed that needle aspiration, controlled by the scanner: (a) will reduce intracranial pressure by a considerable and verifiable amount, and (b) that its efficiency is enhanced by the accuracy and selectivity of antibiotic treatment. Out of 13 cases, treated by needle aspiration and an association of 'penicillin and metronidazole' or 'chloramphenicol and gentalline', they have only observed one death, the others having recovered with no sequelae. Needling only had to be repeated in one case, and excision was only necessary once because of the thickness of the wall.

In regard to the otologist's attitude, Vaneecloo et al. [246] have analyzed 25 cases of otogenic abscesses, observed between 1975 and

1980, with a mortality rate of 8%. In this series, the neurosurgical attitude was to carry out, in the same operation, needling followed by removal of the mass. The authors attribute their good results to the fact that ENT surgery was carried out as soon as possible after the neurosurgery. Two weeks appeared to them to be too long, given the relatively trouble-free nature of the ear operation which could be carried out on a patient whose neurological condition still gave cause for concern. In fact, in every case, they observed a zone of localized meningitis and the abscess had spread by contiguity. It is necessary to eliminate the seat as soon as possible as it is a source of reinfection. In any event, whichever attitude is adopted, these figures show a clear improvement over the statistics from the 1960s when the mortality rate was around 25%.

Cholesteatoma Surgery

General

The aim of all cholesteatoma surgery is complete removal of the cholesteatoma. This explains why for long the only technique used was that of opening all the middle cavities and why, for some, it is still the safest method of eradicating a cholesteatoma. Nowadays, in fact, most otologists, when they are obliged to carry out a radical mastoidectomy, complete the operation by 'management of the tympanic cavity', thus carrying out an open-cavity tympanoplasty. This technique has been given the name, by some authors, including Portmann [169, 170], of 'open technique' as opposed to 'closed technique'. This too aims at complete eradication of the cholesteatoma while preserving the external auditory which has two advantages: it avoids any pathology which is peculiar to the mastoid cavity, and it reconstructs the ossicular chain, keeping the anatomical structure as close to normal as possible.

We shall therefore define, together with the advantages and disadvantages of each, radical mastoidectomy, open-technique tympanoplasty, and closed-technique tympanoplasty. We have decided not to consider such partial operations as atticotomy, atticoantrostomy or partial mastoidectomy since, in our view at least, the mastoid must be treated in an 'all-or-nothing' way; we disapprove strongly of the so-called 'as required' or 'from in front backward' technique.

Radical Mastoidectomy

This is the complete removal of the cholesteatoma, at the price of sacrificing the whole external auditory canal, as described by Stacke in 1890; the technique consists of joining the tympanic cavity and the mastoid into one single cavity. It is thus hoped to achieve complete epidermization of the cavity. For this to be satisfactory, adequate aera-

tion is required. Such a cavity is the result of the (radical) mastoidectomy, or more recently 'canal wall down' technique ('évidement petro-
mastoïdien' in French, and 'Radikal Operation' in German).

Advantages and Disadvantages

Advantages. This technique is generally accepted as safe for the
following reasons: (a) the existence of an open cavity protects against
recurrence of the cholesteatoma, at least if it is adequately aerated, and
(b) even should there be a recurrence, it would be less serious because
it can be detected quickly and because, even when not kept under observation, the lack of any barrier to exteriorization reduces the risk of
any serious complication. We, however, are in fact of the same view as
Marquet and Bremond in that exteriorized and inflamed epidermis in
contact with the bone seems to present a greater potential for invasion
than a cholesteatoma pearl found during the course of second look at a
chronic otitis media with cholesteatoma which has been operated on
using the closed-technique, since the bone-eroding action of the Malpighian tissue in fact depends to a large extent on the inflammation of
the epidermis.

Disadvantages. The main disadvantage of this type of surgery,
which 'sacrifices the mucosa to the skin' [26], is the need for constant,
life-long follow-up and inspection of the mastoidectomy cavity. This
cavity may become the seat of (a) blockage by cerumen or skin, which
may be infected or not, or (b) of suppuration originating in the Eustachian tube. To avoid this pathology, which appears to be relatively
common, we shall describe techniques for creating this mastoidectomy
cavity more successfully. Another disadvantage which affects the patient's comfort is the danger of water entering the ear, with a risk of
infection, vertigo and otalgia. One last disadvantage may be severe
deafness, which is a common but not inevitable sequela of radical mastoidectomy.

Open-Technique Tympanoplasty

This is very similar to radical mastoidectomy, the only difference
being 'management of the tympanic cavity', assuming of course that

the cholesteatoma appears to have been completely removed. By 'management of the tympanic cavity', we mean either simply closing it, or closing the cavity and creating a modified columellar effect ('modified radical mastoidectomy').

Advantages and Disadvantages

Advantages. In addition to the theoretical advantages attached to radical mastoidectomy, which we have already seen, other advantages are linked to the closure of the tympanic cavity. The mucosa of the Eustachian tube and the tympanic cavity is placed in a physiological situation which prevents suppuration originating in the Eustachian tube, which is often found in mastoid cavities, and epidermization of the tympanic cavity which makes it difficult to make any subsequent attempt to restore function. Furthermore, this open-technique tympanoplasty may improve hearing.

Disadvantages. In addition to the disadvantages attached to radical mastoidectomy, there is the risk of a residual cholesteatoma developing in a closed tympanic cavity. It is however only relatively serious, as it is generally easy to detect. In any event, whether the operation is a radical mastoidectomy or an open-technique tympanoplasty, a large cavity must very often be managed by meatoconchoplasty, by obliteration or by a combination of the two procedures. The skin is obviously made to cover the outside of the body. If it is on the inside of a cavity, it is pathological unless there is adequate aeration. It will desquamate and macerate, and there will be hyperplasia of the deeper layers. It may even turn into a cholesteatoma matrix. It thus appears to be of fundamental importance to maintain a satisfactory balance between the surface area of the skin within the cavity and the volume of air circulating at its surface. In fact, this ratio varies from one individual to another and for a variety of reasons – individual factors such as life-style, for example. To sum up, when a very large cavity has been created, there is a risk that the skin which covers it will be inadequately aerated and one of the following courses of action should be taken; increasing aeration by meatoplasty or even conchoplasty; partially reducing the size of the cavity by obliteration; or combining the two procedures.

Closed-Technique Tympanoplasty

Definition

This is a transmastoid approach to the cholesteatoma carried out in such a way that the entire external auditory canal is preserved. After removal, this technique makes it easy to close the tympanic cavity by a new tympanic membrane and to reconstruct the ossicular chain in the same operation or at some subsequent stage. This technique necessarily involves a posterior tympanotomy – also known as 'intact canal wall technique', 'canal wall up', or a 'combined approach tympanoplasty' (CAT).

The posterior tympanotomy is a window created between the tympanic sulcus and the facial nerve, medial and posterior to the former, and lateral and anterior to the latter. Its usefulness is fourfold: (1) It is the only technique which will allow the removal of a cholesteatoma extension, or of an epidermization which is so often encountered in the facial recess which may indeed be the only seat of these lesions. It may be extended downwards as required to cure lesions of the hypotympanum. (2) It allows, even when the bony canal is preserved, exploration of the windows and removal of any lesions which may have their seat there. (3) It represents a ventilation and drainage canal, rendered necessary by the volume of the mastoid cavity which requires a greater volume or air circulating within it. (4) Lastly, it makes it possible to check, up to the final phase of the closed-tympanic operation, the stability of the reconstruction of the ossicular chain.

Advantages and Disadvantages

Advantages. In a general way, these can be said to make for a more comfortable life than can be obtained by the open technique. Unlike the open techniques, the patient is not obliged to submit to regular checks to clean his cavity. The fact of having a closed tympanic cavity avoids any risk attached to water entering the ear. Hearing, which is often adequate for social purposes, also contributes to a more pleasant life.

Disadvantages. These are of two kinds: (1) The first is the risk of a residual cholesteatoma, which is both commoner and more serious. It is commoner because insufficiently eradicated from certain areas which are particularly difficult to set at: this is true of the facial recess, which should be routinely opened during posterior tympanotomy, of the anterior part of the attic, and of the supra-tubal recess, which should be opened into the mesotympanum and the tube, whereas the sinus tympani is always out of sight. It is more serious because it often develops unsuspected within a large antro-atticomastoid cavity and behind a new tympanic membrane which will remain intact long term. It can thus be revealed only when complications occur. These factors explain why we, like most authors, routinely include a second stage: a second look or 'revision'. This second look may make it possible to improve hearing. The only differences are in the timing, but most agree on the interval of 12–18 months. (2) The other disadvantage is the risk of true recurrence of the cholesteatoma. By true recurrence of the cholesteatoma we mean the recurrence of a retraction pocket, which is known to be a most common mechanism by which cholesteatoma originates. But we have various devices for preventing, by mechanical means which have their limits, recurrence of these pockets:

(a) Reconstruction of the bony sulcus must keep as close as possible to the normal anatomical structure, since it is known that the slightest loss of substance, particularly from the attic wall, can favour a retraction pocket. It may even be necessary to reduce the size of the tympanic frame in order to make the tympanic membrane smaller and thus reduce the risk of a retraction pocket.

(b) The texture of some materials used to repair the tympanic membrane may help prevent the recurrence of a retraction pocket. Perichondrium and tympanic membrane homografts, because of their radial structure, are thought to be the best materials by some of the present authors.

(c) Partial obliteration of the attic may be done – either by leaving the remaining parts of the other ossicles in place when they are healthy, or, if they are not, by replacing them by other ossicles in a total tympano-ossicular homograft. For some of the present authors, this seems to be the ideal solution.

(d) Insertion of a sheet of Silastic, by preventing the development of fibrosis, is also a means of avoiding the appearance of a retraction pocket, associated with such fibrotic adhesions.

(e) For some surgeons, including Portmann [169, 170], a posterior tympanotomy, especially if large, may favour the appearance of a retraction pocket leading to the recurrence of a cholesteatoma. They therefore close it, partially or totally, at the end of the operation.

The use of these techniques is in our opinion essential to the success of closed-technique tympanoplasty. We are nonetheless aware that they are only devices which can relieve, by mechanical means, a dysfunction of the Eustachian tube, many physiological and pathological aspects of which are still unfortunately unknown to us. The following are also to be considered together with closed techniques: temporary removal of the posterosuperior wall of the external auditory canal during surgery, 'removing and replacing' the canal – this is attractive in theory but may in practice lead to some difficulty [67, 68]; or removal and replacement of the attic wall [259].

Operative Procedure

We shall not deal exhaustively with this since it would involve a description of the whole of otological surgery, but we shall particularly emphasize those techniques concerned with: (a) the eradication of a cholesteatoma wherever it may be located, so as to avoid any residual cholesteatoma, and (b) the prevention of true recurrence through retraction pockets, which are often favoured by Eustachian tube malfunction, and which should be dealt with by the devices mentioned above. We shall not thus go into any detail on the types of anaesthetic to be used, except to stress the advantage in using an associated local anaesthetic to reduce bleeding and make the elevation of the skin of the external auditory meatus easier.

Radical Mastoidectomy

Approaches

All the different approaches give proper access to the cavities of the middle ear, and it is in fact each surgeon's individual habits which will determine the choice of approach used. We shall give a brief description of the four main approaches:

(1) The Endaural Incision and Its Variations

The vertical incision is made between the helix and the tragus, and is 1 or 2 cm in length, although it may be extended higher in the ex-

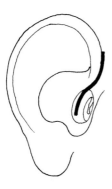 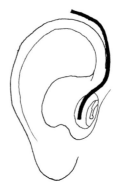

Fig. 35. Endaural incision.
Fig. 36. Extended Fleury endaural incision.

tended endaural incision [77]. The horizontal incision is made at the point where the cartilaginous canal and the bony canal join, and goes from 8 o'clock round to 2 o'clock on a right ear. For some surgeons this is the most logical approach, since it gives direct access to the cavities of the middle ear and, more especially, because it automatically involves a meatoplasty. For others it is inadequate when the mastoid cavity is large, since it may not permit complete exposure of such a cavity, particularly towards the tip (fig. 35, 36).

(2) Posterior Incision and Its Variations

The skin incision may be made in the posterior sulcus itself (Portmann's posterosuperior incision – fig. 37) [505] or continue beyond it posteriorly, cutting a flap which is purely cutaneous posteriorly, and cutaneomuscular anteriorly (Marquet's incision – fig. 38). If a Palva's flap is desired, the musculoperiosteal flap must be adequately incised; the technique will be described in detail further on.

(3) Heermann's Incision

This is an extended endaural incision, continued beyond the auricle into the postaural region about as far as the level of the middle of the auricle (fig. 39). It is thus very similar to Fleury's extended endaural incision.

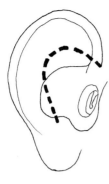 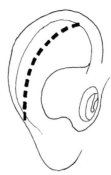

Fig. 37. Portmann's posterosuperior incision.
Fig. 38. Marquet's skin incision.

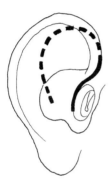 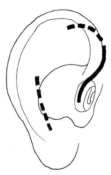

Fig. 39. Heermann's extended incision continuing into the postaural region.
Fig. 40. Combined approach: extended endaural incision with inferior postaural incision.

(4) Combined Approaches

These are a combination of: either an extended endaural incision and an inferior postaural incision (fig. 40) – (Fleury et al. [77] use this combination when the mastoid pathology is greatly extended posteriorly or in a particularly large tip; or a standard postaural incision and a limited endaural incision (fig. 41); or a posteriorly displaced postaural incision of the Marquet type, and an incision transfixing the canal at the base of the mastoid cortex (fig. 42).

Bonework

The antro-atticomastoidectomy sacrifices the posterosuperior wall of the external bony auditory canal. It involves: enlargement of the bony external auditory meatus, centred on the spine of Henle, thinning of the lateral bony wall of the antrum and attic in order to create a step, opening the cavities, the size of the cavity being related to the extent of the lesions and the pneumatization of the mastoid, removal of the bony bridge making up the lower edge of the attic wall. The most important points are to ensure total eradication of the cholesteatoma and to ensure that the definitive operative cavity is aerated, drained and easy to inspect, which presupposes that precise criteria as regards the size and management of the posterior cavity will be observed.

Eradication of the Cholesteatoma Itself

In the Antrum and Mastoid Cavity. The general principle is to remove the cholesteatoma from behind forward. But there are different problems depending on whether the mastoid is sclerotic or, on the contrary, more or less pneumatized, especially in children. When the mastoid is sclerotic, the matrix of the cholesteatoma hernial sac is easily separated from the underlying tissue with an elevator and suction. When, on the other hand, the mastoid is still pneumatized, the whole cellular system must be opened in order to make a systematic search for any extension of a large cholesteatoma. This removal of the complete cell system is in any event necessary to prevent the remaining, insufficiently aerated, mucosa from causing lesions of the cholesterol granuloma type.

In the Attic. Here the cholesteatoma must be removed from in front backward and from above downward. It is always possible, during these manoeuvres, that the surgeon may discover, either the lateral sinus or the dura mater, exposed over a surface which varies from case to case, or more particularly, a dehiscent facial nerve, this being most common in the second portion and at the genu in the case of a cholesteatoma in the attic and antrum. In the region of the lateral semicircular canal, the surgeon must be especially meticulous in his search for a fistula. He should use suction to remove the squames from a matrix covering the canal, palpate such a matrix with a blunt needle to detect any depression, and make a careful search for any correspondence

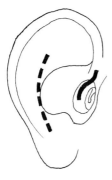 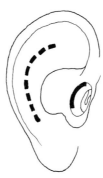

Fig. 41. Standard postaural incision combined with a limited endaural incision.

Fig. 42. Combined approach: posteriorly displaced postaural incision combined with an incision transfixing the canal.

with the oval window. We shall describe the strictly technical aspects of the dissection of such a fistula further on. In any event, the cholesteatoma must be dissected with great care and meticulous detail.

In the Mesotympanum. It is often very difficult to dissect the cholesteatoma because its seat may be difficult or even impossible to get at, and also because of the state of the mucosa. This, however, is where the real advantage of the radical mastoidectomy lies – in allowing some remnants of cholesteatoma matrix to be left in these regions, with, of course, regular follow-up and inspection. It is, on the other hand, necessary to excise the cholesteatoma completely from the mesotympanum when an open-technique tympanoplasty has been decided upon, and we shall return to this difficulty in due course. During the operation, such an excision involves the sacrifice of the remaining parts of the tympanic membrane and ossicles.

Creation of the Posterior Cavity

Certain technical criteria must be observed if it is wished to avoid those complications, specific to such a cavity, which have partially discredited radical mastoidectomy. The aim is to create a cavity which is theoretically self-cleansing, i.e. a cavity which is permanently cicatrized with spontaneous evacuation of squamous tissue towards the meatus. The various criteria are: total removal of the facial ridge, drilling away of all the mastoid cell tracts, elimination of all overhangs,

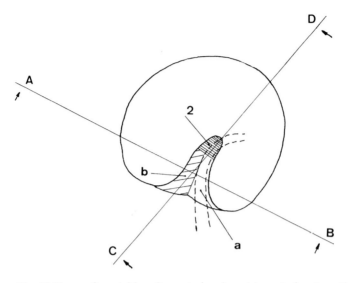

Fig. 43. Shape of mastoid cavity: anterior slope (a), posterior slope (b), and posterior buttress (2).

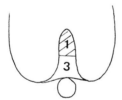

Fig. 44. A–B cross section showing height of facial ridge: superficial zone (1) and deep dangerous zone (3).

especially in the anterior part of the attic and the tip of the mastoid, proper shaping of the edges of the cavity.

Total Removal of the Facial Ridge. The objective to be attained is the lowering of the facial ridge as far as the horizontal plane passing through the inferior wall of the external bony auditory canal, in order to eliminate any ledge between the antromastoid cavity and the floor of the meatus. The result of this lowering is to change the kidney-

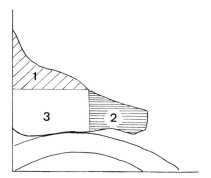

Fig. 45. Diagram of facial ridge (C–D cross section): superficial zone (1), posterior buttress (2), and deep zone (3).

shaped cavity into a rounded, almost circular cavity. Only the tip lies inevitably below the floor of the canal. This is an essential precondition for satisfactory drainage and ventilation, and for effective follow-up and inspection.

Technique: After the attic, antrum and mastoid cavity have been opened, the facial ridge appears as a bony protuberance in the shape of a pyramid, with an inferior base and a superior summit, or posterior buttress, separating the antrum and the mastoid from behind from the tympanic cavity in front (fig. 43, 44), bisecting the cavity. The facial ridge has an anterior slope, a posterior slope, and a lateral portion. These are the three portions which must be thinned away until contact is made with the facial canal.

Fleury et al. [78] divide the facial canal ridge into three zones. The removal of the superficial peripheral zone is easy and relatively danger-free. In the limited zone of the posterior buttress and the facial recess, standard procedure is never to go deeper than a plane passing through the dome of the lateral semicircular canal. The removal of the deep dangerous zone is the most difficult, and indeed the most trying step. Its anterior slope corresponds to the 'overhang' or 'triangular fold' of the facial ridge. An angled probe will give an idea of the size of this overhang, which must be lowered very carefully because of the possible proximity of the facial nerve. Its posterior slope corresponds to the most anterior part of the cell tract between the facial nerve and the sigmoid sinus (fig. 43). Its middle part is the most difficult step.

Progress must be slow, with constant reference to nearby anatomical landmarks (fig. 45).

In fact, in our opinion, the second portion of the facial nerve, which is easily identifiable above the oval window, its angle indicating the probable location of the third portion, seems to be the best landmark, which should be taken into consideration for the whole of the third portion. Another way to get round the problems caused by the frequent variations in the path of the facial nerve is to identify the third portion of the facial nerve in its hard bone. These three portions of the facial ridge are lowered simultaneously, using medium-sized multi-toothed burrs. Drilling should always to be carried out parallel to the facial nerve. As soon as the bone starts to become harder, the facial canal is near and diamond burrs should be used. The risk of injury to the nerve is greatest in the lower part of the third portion.

Drilling Away All the Mastoid Cell Tracts. This drilling away of all the cell tracts (above and behind the labyrinth, in the sinodural angle, between the facial nerve and the sigmoid sinus, at the tip of the mastoid and behind the sinus) is necessary in order to avoid the production of inflammatory granulation tissue. Drilling must continue until the white, relatively homogeneous and dense bone of the cortex is reached. At the end of this drilling, the surgeon should be able to run his forefinger over a perfectly smooth surface, especially around the tip of the mastoid.

Elimination of All Overhangs. It is essential to exenterate the anterior buttress of the attic so that its anterior wall is flush with the anterior wall of the external auditory canal, and to exenterate the tip of the mastoid, which may contain cells with cholesterol granuloma or osteitis.

Proper Shaping of the Edge of the Cavity. The edges of the cavity should be cut to a gentle slope wherever possible (zone behind the sinus and the tip of the mastoid) in order to reduce the volume of the operation cavity by natural joining of the soft tissues (Paparella's 'saucerization') [478].

Management of the Mastoid Cavity

It must be remembered that the management of the mastoid cavity must seek to maintain a satisfactory ratio between the area of skin lin-

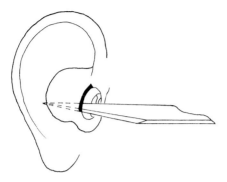

Fig. 46. Meatoplasty; transfixing incision.

ing the cavity and the volume of free air in contact with its surface. It is therefore possible, when the cavity is large, either to increase the ventilation by enlarging the meatus, or to reduce the size of the cavity by obliteration to a greater or lesser extent. If these rules are not observed, there is the risk of the appearance of pathology in the cavity itself, and especially of the recurrence of a cholesteatoma. This is why we stress the importance of this type of procedure, which can avoid such problems. We shall therefore describe meatoplasty and obliteration of the mastoid cavity.

Meatoplasty. The type of meatoplasty will be chosen according to the size of the cavity which is to be aerated and inspected. The axis of the meatoplasty must also coincide with the large axis of the cavity to ensure maximum ventilation and easy inspection. We shall therefore describe three techniques:

(1) The easiest to carry out, when an endaural incision has been used, is a simple opening between the tragus and the helix.

(2) When a posterior approach has been used, a meatoplasty with no removal of cartilage is also simple to carry out. It is similar to a standard T-shaped meatoplasty. *First step:* an incision is made transfixing the canal skin in the meatus, from 12 o'clock to 6 o'clock (fig. 46). *Second step:* two counter-incisions are made at the upper and

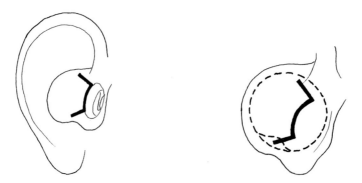

Fig. 47, 48. Superior and inferior counterincisions.

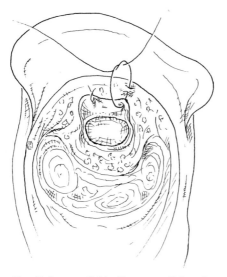

Fig. 49. Suture of skin flap to medial surface of concha.

lower limits of the first incision. The radical mastoidectomy cavity must be adequately exposed (fig. 47, 48). *Third step:* the resulting skin flap is sutured to the posterior surface of the conchal cartilage, which has previously been thinned (fig. 49). *Fourth step:* the remaining canal skin is incised in a manner which varies from author to author; the flap or flaps are thinned then placed against the bony wall of the cavity so as to initiate its epidermization (fig. 50–53).

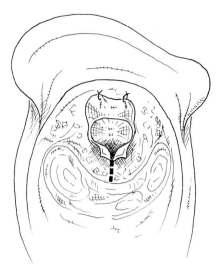

Fig. 50. Posterior incision of skin of external auditory meatus.

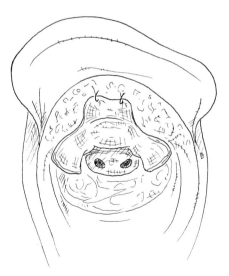

Fig. 51. Flaps in place after posterior incision of canal skin.

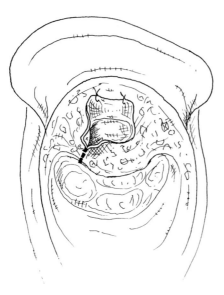

Fig. 52. Superior incision with inferiorly based flap of skin from external auditory meatus.

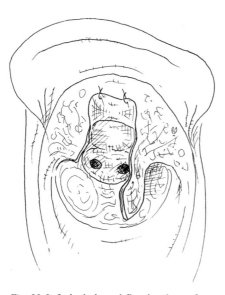

Fig. 53. Inferiorly based flap in place after superior incision of canal skin.

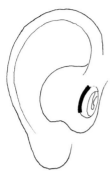

Fig. 54. Large Y-shaped Siebenmann meatoplasty-transfixing incision.

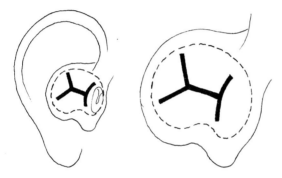

Fig. 55, 56. Y-shaped incision of conchal cartilage.

(3) Large Y-shaped Siebenmann-type meatoplasty with removal of cartilage. This meatoplasty is very rarely used. *First step:* the canal skin is transfixed, using the same incision as for the previous operation (fig. 54). *Second step:* a Y-shaped incision is made in the conchal cartilage: the upright should be incised so as to pass through the centre line of the mastoid cavity (fig. 55, 56). The lengths of the two other limbs will depend on the size of the cavity. Three skin-cartilage flaps have now been created. *Third step:* the three triangles of cartilage are removed so that only the skin is retained (fig. 57, 58). *Fourth step:* the remaining part of the canal skin is incised in different ways by differ-

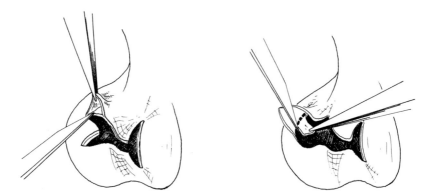

Fig. 57, 58. Removal of triangles of cartilage.

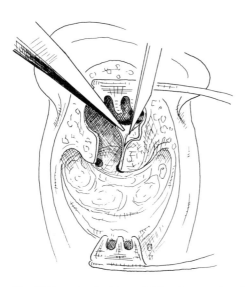

Fig. 59. Posterior incision of skin of external auditory meatus.

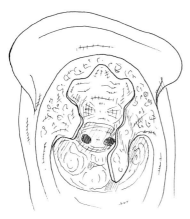

Fig. 60. Superior incision to create inferiorly based flap.

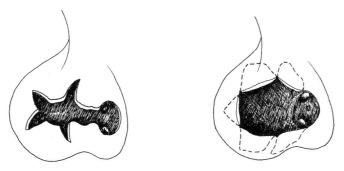

Fig. 61. Appearances of the five meatoplasty skin flaps.
Fig. 62. Final positioning of five meatoplasty skin flaps.

ent authors, as in the last technique (fig. 59, 60). *Fifth step:* the three flaps from the concha and the flap or flaps from the meatus are placed so as to initiate the epithelialization of the cavity (fig. 61, 62).

Meatoconchoplasty, finally, is used by most authors when there is a large cavity in order to improve ventilation and make inspection easier. It must however be remembered how important the method of creating the cavity is, and in particular that the edges should be shaped to form a gentle slope, allowing a considerable reduction in the surface area of the operation cavity, and thus rendering a large meatoplasty unnecessary. But it must be borne in mind, on the other hand, that despite these unquestionable advantages, there is a risk of perichondritis developing if the operation is carried out in particularly septic conditions. Lastly, the unattractive appearance of a large meatoplasty must not be forgotten.

Obliteration. The aim here is to reduce the size of the mastoid cavity and thus the surface to be aerated. The majority of authors only advise its use with the utmost caution in cases of cholesteatoma. Their fear is that a cholesteatoma may recur unseeen beneath the obliteration. Only when it is absolutely certain that the cholesteatoma has been completely eradicated can this solution be contemplated in cases where the mastoid cavity is large.

Different types of material may be described. Musculoperiosteal-fascial flaps are the most commonly used; their pedicle may be posterior, anterosuperior, anterior or inferior. Free grafts of subcutaneous periosteal tissue may be used, bone or cartilage grafts used alone or together, or synthetic substances, such as proplast, teflon, ceramics, osseine or silicone. These would seem to be experiments which we have culled from the literature on the subject, but their results should be interpreted with great care.

Quite apart from the possibility that they may mask the recurrence of a cholesteatoma, these obliterations have their own disadvantages. In the short term, infection is a contra-indication when the cavity is particularly septic. In such cases, several of the present authors will only adopt such a solution secondarily after halting the infection. In the long term, resorption, even if it is only partial, is a frequent problem. Nevertheless, obliteration may be used as a tympanoplasty procedure as we well see later.

Combined Techniques. These combine both meatoplasty and obliteration, but are in fact rarely used, since most authors are reluctant to obliterate the cavity in cases of chronic otitis media with cholesteatoma especially noted by a radical mastoidectomy.

Closure of the Eustachian Tube. This has been suggested by some authors. They use free muscle grafts placed in the tubal orifice and the protympanum.

Complete Exclusion

This technique has been proposed by Rambo, Gacek [85] and by Montandon and Smoli [147]. It involves a particularly thorough radical mastoidectomy – all the remaining skin and mucosa must be removed. Obliteration is carried out, either with a muscle flap or with adipose tissue – each has its proponents. The operation involves the sacrifice of the canal skin, or at least of its medial portion, since, on the surface, the anterior and posterior flaps are sutured so as to exclude the middle ear. For these authors, the indications, although rare, may concern certain patients who have been operated on several occasions, who are partially or totally deaf and who wish to lead a normal life without the problems caused by the introduction of water into the ear. Obviously, such operations are not without risk in cases of chronic otitis media with cholesteatoma.

Open-Technique Tympanoplasty

This, as we have said, is a radical mastoidectomy, the cavity being closed by a new tympanic membrane with or without the reconstruction of a columellar effect. The closure of the tympanic cavity has three advantages. It prevents epithelialization, which could be a major barrier to any subsequent attempt to improve function. It disposes of the risk of otorrhea of the Eustachian tube, a fairly common occurrence when the cavity remains open during a radical mastoidectomy. Hearing may improve. But it can obviously only be carried out if the tympanic cavity was free from cholesteatoma. If there had been invasion by the cholesteatoma, the surgeon must be absolutely sure that eradication has been complete. We shall therefore look first at the techniques for complete removal of the cholesteatoma from the tympanic cavity, and then at those for the management of the cavity itself. We shall only consider these two steps of the operation in any detail, as the approaches, the removal of the cholesteatoma from the antro-atticomastoid cavity, and the drilling of the cavity are in every way identical to those we have already described for radical mastoidectomy. The only possible difference could be the Palva-type obliteration of the posterior cavity with muscle tissue, which is frequently practised by one of the present authors. This technique will be described further on.

Removal of the Cholesteatoma from the Tympanic Cavity
There is often great difficulty in dissecting the cholesteatoma, because its seat may be difficult or even impossible to get at, or because

of the state of the mucosa. The general principle is to push the choles-teatoma away from the peripheral area towards the windows which must be dissected at the last stage in the eradication. The cholestea-toma may extend peripherally to the facial recess, the hypotympanum, the Eustachian tube, or the anterior attic. But in practice, there is al-most always at least one healthy area from which to begin the dissec-tion.

Even with an open technique, on the other hand, there may be great difficulty in dissecting a cholesteatoma in the region of the facial recess, and particularly around the sinus tympani, and also around the Eustachian tube [178]. In the region of the sinus tympani, every effort must be made to ensure that the dissection can be carried out with visual control. The operating table should be tipped as far as possible towards the surgeon, who should use mirrors, resect the pyramid, and the whole of the anterior slope of the facial ridge. Despite the ma-noeuvres, and despite the use of an open technique, the dissection is all too often carried out without visual control, simply by contact. Every effort must be made not to break the matrix if removal is to be com-plete.

An extension of the cholesteatoma to the Eustachian tube may likewise turn out to be impossible to extract if it is of any size, since only the first few millimetres of the superior lateral wall of the tube can be drilled, because of the risk of damage to the internal carotid. Around the windows which, as we have said, are to be dissected at the end of the operation in order to minimize the possible risk of traumatic lesions and their consequences, the surgeon must take great pains to avoid damaging the secondary tympanic membrane of the round win-dow, or the superstructure or footplate of the stapes. The manoeuvres will be described in detail in the section on the closed technique. The state of the mucosa of the tympanic cavity is important in deter-mining the difficulty involved in dissecting the cholesteatoma. Dis-section is generally easy when the mucosa is oedematous, but practi-cally impossible when he mucosa is dry and atrophied to a greater or lesser extent, making it necessary for the surgeon to sacrifice it as required.

Management of the Tympanic Cavity

We shall describe the closure of the tympanic cavity and the recon-struction of the columella.

Closure of the Tympanic Cavity

Several situations are possible. The pars tensa may be intact. In this case, a fascia graft is slid under its medial surface, resting on the second portion of the facial canal. There may be no useable remnants of the tympanic membrane. In this case, a myringoplasty may be carried out using a fascia graft resting anteriorly and posteriorly on the sulcus and superiorly and posteriorly on the facial canal. If the eradication of the cholesteatoma, or more precisely of the squamous epithelium, has involved removal of the mucosa to any extent, some of the present authors line the mesotympanum, with a thick sheet of silastic if it is intended to reconstruct the columella during a second operation, when it will be removed. In practice, the limited depth of these cavities does not always allow the use of thick silastic. A thin sheet of silastic is used, if it is intended to reconstruct the columella immediately, but it must be pointed out that such a sheet, because of its very thinness, may roll up and thus prove ineffective. The essential role of the silastic is in fact to ensure satisfactory regeneration of the mucosa from remainings islands of healthy tissue, usually to be found near the orifice of the Eustachian tube, by counteracting fibrosis, which would negate any positive result by the resultant adhesions. These adhesions are all the more to be avoided because, with an open-technique tympanoplasty, the cavity is not deep. This factor also explains the occasional exteriorization of the silastic.

Reconstruction of the Columella

This may be carried out immediately or during a second stage. If the stapes is intact, the surgeon may carry out a simple myringostapediopexy or may build up the stapes. If the superstructure is absent, some authors will use their own individual method to reconstruct the columella, with the added advantage that the graft is prevented from sinking on to the promontory.

In the final analysis, the prognosis of these open-technique tympanoplasties is governed by: (a) the extent to which the mucosa is sacrificed: this is why the use of silastic is advantageous, although, as we have pointed out, there is the risk of its elimination in shallow tympanic cavities; (b) the effectiveness of the aeration through the Eustachian tube: any dysfunction will favour retraction with a risk of symphysis; (c) the shallowness of the tympanic cavity: some of the present authors therefore, in order to give proper depth to the cavity, set up a

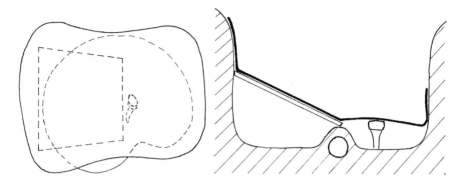

Fig. 63, 64. Setting up a superior 'console' to support the graft.

sort of superior 'console' (fig. 63, 64), with bone or cartilage grafts; the aim is to achieve a true open-technique tympanoplasty immediately.

Obliteration of the Posterior Cavity

Some of the present authors carry out a fibromuscular obliteration [33, 34, 42, 61] using Palva's flap [160].

Skin incision: it should be made posteriorly, more than usual, then continue anteriorly (fig. 65). The skin and the subcutaneous tissue are elevated over the whole surface of the mastoid as far as the tip inferiorly and the cartilaginous canal anteriorly (fig. 66).

Cutting the flap: the incision of the musculoperiosteal covering should be made as posteriorly as possible and continue superiorly along the inferior edge of the temporal muscle as far as the line perpendicular to the anterior wall of the external auditory meatus. The flap is then detached from the bone with an electric knife and the fibromuscular covering of the tip is elevated, creating a flap with an anterior hinge which, at the end of the operation, will fall naturally into the posterior cavity to form the posterior portion of the new canal (fig. 66).

Drilling the cavity: the bony canal is eliminated and the cavity is drilled as regular as a properly executed mastoidectomy: complete lowering of facial ridge, removal of the anterior buttress, saucerization of the mastoid bowl in order to reduce the space to be obliterated.

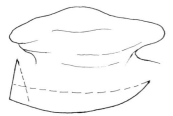

Fig. 65. Palva's flap: posterosuperior skin incision and resection for traction meato-plasty.

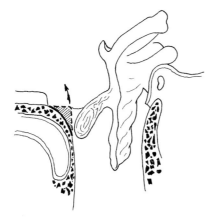

Fig. 66. Palva's flap: anteriorly hinged muscle flap.

Reconstruction: the tympanic membrane is reconstructed usually with fascia in underlay. The obliteration is carried out by free fibro-muscular grafts in attic and antrum covered by the fibromuscular flap. The fascia graft rests on the flap. The canal skin finally is folded back over the flap and the graft. If the tympanic cavity is pathological and has to be dissected, thin or thick silastic is left under the graft so as to prevent the symphysis of the tympanic cavity. If the cavity is healthy, the ossicular chain may be reconstructed at once and in such cases this type of tympanoplasty can be carried out in a single operation (fig. 67).

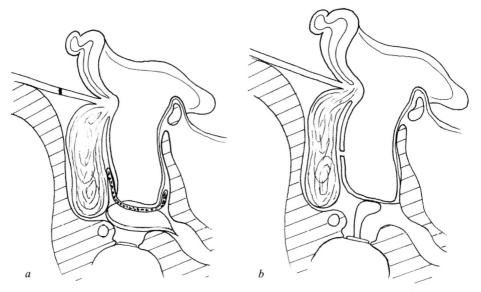

Fig. 67. Open-technique tympanoplasty with obliteration by a Palva's fibromuscular flap: *a* end of the 1st stage (upper segment of horizontal section); *b* end of the 2nd stage (upper segment of horizontal section).

Meatoplasty: this comprises three steps, two at the beginning of the process, one at its end. A skin resection of a part of posterosuperior approach is performed (fig. 65). An incision is made between the tragus and the helix as in the vertical part of Shambaugh's incision, but starting from the sulcus at the level of the malleus. This incision also divides the muscle tissue to delineate the anterior limit of the fibromuscular flap. Soft tissue covering the anterior buttress is removed. At the end of the operation, a strong, slightly tense suture on two levels will open the incision between the tragus and the helix, performing a 'traction meatoplasty'.

Second stage: if a second stage is indicated, it is usually performed by a transmeatal approach. The tympanic cavity is opened by cutting a tympanoparietal flap, overlapping into the muscle obliteration. The tympanic cavity can easily be identified by following the canal floor. The silastic is removed. If there is a residual pearl, it can be removed. The ossicular chain is reconstructed in healthy mucosa and between a stable tympanic membrane and the stapes or the footplate (fig. 67).

The flap itself is rarely and only partially lifted during this second stage. The posterior approach is used to lift the flap from the mastoid, antrum and aditus. It is very important to leave the flap attached to the external semicircular canal and area of the mastoid part of facial nerve. Lifting totally this flap could cause it to atrophy. In fact, the risk of inclusion of skin behind the flap must be minimized or suppressed by taking great care in the surgical technique with additional dissection and bonework.

Closed Techniques

Approaches

Posterior incisions and their variations are in our view the only incisions appropriate to an antro-atticomastoidectomy using a transmastoid route which is sufficiently enlarged superiorly and posteriorly to permit a successful posterior tympanotomy. To carry out a posterior tympanotomy, an oblique angle is necessary, and since this is only obtainable by a posterior approach, the endaural incision must be rejected because of its limitations.

Transmastoid Antro-Atticomastoidectomy

Initial Drilling. A large burr is used to drill within a triangle limited: anteriorly by the posterosuperior wall of the external auditory meatus as far as the root of the zygoma, superiorly be the linea temporalis and posteriorly by a line, about 3 cm from the posterior meatal wall, between the sinodural angle and the tip of the mastoid.

Drilling and Opening the Cavities. Wide sweeps are made over the bone surface using a large burr. Anteriorly, the posterosuperior meatal wall should be sculptured so that a constant adequate thickness is preserved throughout, and so that the endaural and mastoid sides are strictly parallel. Some of the present authors remodel the endaural slope of this wall in order to obtain a better view, especially of its lower portion (fig. 68). It is very important that this wall should be constantly kept in view, so that it can be kept intact.

Posteriorly, the surgeon must watch for the bluish colour of the lateral sinus, and superiorly, the pinkish colour of the meninges. The

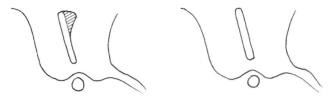

Fig. 68. Remodelling the endaural portion of the posterior wall of the external auditory meatus.

antrum is opened, then enlarged inferiorly and posteriorly as required. Anteriorly, it is enlarged towards the attic, using a smaller burr and working by contact with the posterosuperior meatal wall. Two essential landmarks now appear: the lateral semicircular canal and the short process of the incus. The transmastoid atticotomy is continued anteriorly using even smaller burrs. Drilling is carried out from the deeper level to the more superficial, and the burrs are held so as to follow the curve of the meatus. This avoids any uncovering of the meninges, usually lower anteriorly. In order to avoid any damage, the tegmen and the posterosuperior bony canal wall are skeletonized. The heads of the ossicles have already been exposed. Once this antro-atticomastoidectomy, preserving the bony canal, has been completed, the surgeon must make sure there is no remaining overhang, particularly of the tegmen, anterior attic and lower part of the attic wall.

Posterior Tympanotomy

Two conditions are necessary for the proper execution of the posterior tympanotomy. The antromastoid cavity must be sufficiently enlarged superiorly and posteriorly to permit instruments to be held at the greatest possible angle, and the posterosuperior wall sculptured so as to make the body of the incus, or the fossa incudis when the incus is entirely eroded, completely visible.

Intital drilling is done with small diamond or cutting burrs, following an extension of the line of the short process of the incus by enlarging the fossa incudis inferiorly under continuous irrigation (fig. 69). There is a risk of drilling either too superficially, and nicking the sulcus, or, more especially, too deeply, and damaging the facial nerve. It is also extremely important to avoid any contact between the burr and the incus, to prevent any repercussions in the labyrinth if the

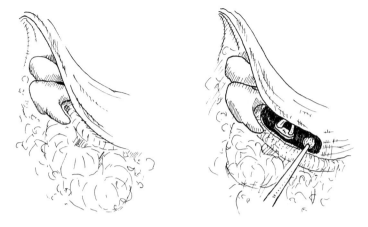

Fig. 69. Exposing the incus and the fossa incudis.

Fig. 70. Posterior tympanotomy: opening the tympanotomy inferiorly, following the facial nerve.

ossicular chains is intact. Two precautionary measures may be taken: either routine dismantling of the incudostapedian joint through the meatus, or the temporary creation of a small bony bridge just behind the incus.

Drilling is done parallel to the facial nerve which is located in its second portion or at the genu – or, for some of the present authors, a systematic search is made for the third portion. Danger of damage of the facial nerve is greatest at the genu, since it is directly subjacent at this point, whereas slightly further down it is posterior and thus protected. At this stage there may occur a problem which will retard the progress of the operation – the discovery of islands of soft tissue which may be hemorrhagic. It is not always easy to distinguish between nerve tissue and cells filled with inflamed mucosa or fibrous tissue ('Angstzellen' in German – Sappey's subadital fossa).

The enlargement towards the hypotympanum is continued as far as is necessary: during the drilling the chorda tympani will be encountered, but its position, in relation to the facial nerve, is not an accurate landmark. It is severed whenever the tympanotomy is extended inferiorly (fig. 70). The posterior tympanotomy thus carried out makes it possible to observe the stapes or its footplate, the pyramidal process and possibly the promontory, the round window and hypotympanum.

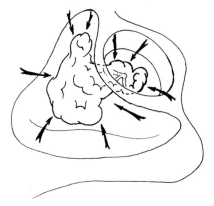

Fig. 71. Removal of cholesteatoma – method.

Removal of the Cholesteatoma Itself

This is done in the same way as was explained for open techniques, i.e., in outline from behind forward in the mastoid cavity, from in front backward and from above downward in the attic, and from the peripheral area towards the windows in the tympanic cavity (fig. 71). But, because the bony canal has been preserved, it is particularly difficult to eradicate a cholesteatoma located in the facial recess, the sinus tympani, the hypotympanum, the anterior attic and the area above the Eustachian tube, the Eustachian tube itself, or the windows. We shall describe those techniques which are best fitted to eradicate the squamous epithelium situated in these areas which are difficult to set at.

Cholesteatoma Located in Facial Recess

This is an extremely common location and may even be the only seat of a cholesteatoma or, even more frequently, of epithelialization. The facial recess lies between the posterior sulcus on its lateral side and the facial nerve on its medial side. It extends downwards as far as the hypotympanum. Pathology in this recess can only be completely eradicated by posterior tympanotomy. After this has been completed, following the procedure we have just detailed, the skin will be removed using a fine suction tip, a hook and a spatula, by the two combined routes – transmastoid and transmeatal.

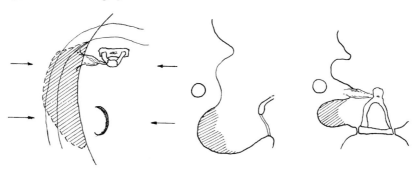

Fig. 72. Diagram showing position of sinus tympani.

Cholesteatoma Located in Sinus Tympani

This too is an extremely common location. It is difficult to eradicate cholesteatomas located here since a large part of the area cannot be visualized. For this reason some surgeons [29, 261, 262] recommend the use of mirrors, but these are often inadequate. Others [78, 196] suggest the removal of the pyramidal process and lowering the anterior slope of the facial ridge as far as possible, but in such devices, although they help to expose the vestibule of the sinus tympani, do not make it possible to get a direct view of the floor of the sinus tympani, and even less of its depths.

One of the present authors, in order to get a better view of this area, uses a speculum to open the meatus, which gives him a more oblique view from in front backwards since he is seated, for this step, opposite the ear on which he is operating. In most cases, therefore, a suitable suction tip is used to detach the skin in block with the mucosa with a large hook or spatula. A small piece of synthetic sponge held with a Marquet forceps may be used for the cleavage of the matrix. If the matrix breaks, it can only be detached 'blind', taking great care not to damage the facial nerve. Although these manoeuvres may be sufficient for the facial recess or a small sinus tympani, they are totally ineffectual for a large sinus tympani with a concealed back portion. One of the present authors therefore suggests opening the sinus tympani to reach its concealed portion. We shall describe the different steps of this operation, but it must be emphasized that it is only indicated when a residual cholesteatoma is discovered during a second look (fig. 72).

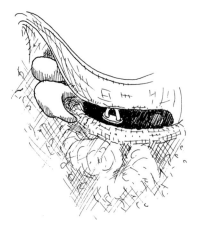

Fig. 73. Opening up the sinus tympani – extension of the posterior tympanotomy towards the round window.

Technique for Opening Up Concealed Portion of Sinus tympani [16, 179]. A posteriorly widened antromastoidectomy, going beyond the lateral sinus, previously skeletonized, is a prerequisite for this technique. This wide cavity makes it possible to incline the burr as near as possible to the plane of the operating table in order to pass the level with the medial face of the facial nerve. The posterior tympanotomy must also have been completed and extended posteriorly until the round window is clearly visible (fig. 73). The round window is an important landmark.

First step: skeletonization of the first part of the third portion of the facial nerve, on its posterior face.

Second step: skeletonization of the lower part of the lateral semicircular canal and of the convexity of the posterior semicircular canal from the point where it crosses the lateral semicircular canal at right angles to its intersection with the facial nerve. This step is perfectly safe on a well pneumatized mastoid, but dangerous on an eburnated mastoid, which will constitute a contraindication. It has the advantage of showing the direction of the posterior semicircular canal which will serve as a landmark during the next step.

Third step: skeletonization of the medial surface of the facial nerve. The starting-point is where the posterior semicircular canal and

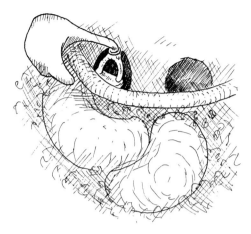

Fig. 74. Opening up the sinus tympani: skeletonization of 3rd portion of facial nerve.

the facial nerve cross. Drilling is done upwards along a line leading from this point to the round window, visible through the posterior tympanotomy (fig. 74). The burr must be held, as far as possible, horizontal in relation to the plane of the headrest, in order to prevent any slipping towards the posterior semicircular canal. If it is impossible to skeletonize the posterior semicircular canal, the starting-point is about 2 mm below the angle formed by the facial nerve and the lateral semicircular canal which is always identifiable.

It must be remembered that this technique is only applicable when there is a large sinus tympani, with a large floor or concealed portion, where there is a considerable risk of a residual cholesteatoma if the surgeon works without visual control. It is this type of sinus tympani which can be opened from the back, since the distance between the facial nerve and the posterior semicircular canal is at least 2 mm.

Cholesteatoma Located in the Hypotympanum

Eradication of a cholesteatoma here involves both a posterior tympanotomy, widened as far as the floor of the bony canal, and a direct approach from the tympanic cavity. The walls between the cells in this region must be drilled away using a diamond burr because of two dangers: (a) the jugular bulb, especially if it is prolapsed, which may, or may not, be convered by a thin bony film, and (b) anteriorly, the internal carotid, which may be affected by the lesions, although only, it is true, in exceptional cases.

The surgeon should move towards the patient's vertex in order to get a better view of this region. At the point where the hypotympanum and the facial recess join, there is another area which may be epithelialized. In some cases it may be necessary to use the same approach route, between the facial nerve and the sigmoid sinus, as is used for glomus jugulare tumours [39], in order to remove this squamous epithelium. This approach may be combined with opening the sinus tympani.

Cholesteatoma Located in the Anterior Attic and the Supra-Tubal Recess

This is one of the most common locations. Total eradication involves an atticotomy, which must be as anterior as possible, and an anterior and superior tympanotomy, opening the anterior attic into the anterosuperior part of the tympanic cavity. Such a tympanotomy therefore, involves the removal of the floor of the region above the Eustachian tube orifice [101]. Eradication is effected simultaneously through the anterior attic and through the tympanic cavity. The surgeon must be extremely careful in the anterior attic to avoid any contact between the burr and the head of the malleus if the ossicular chain is intact. In the vast majority of cases, in fact, the ossicular chain has been interrupted by pathology or surgery. In any event, when the cholesteatoma extends to the anterior attic, the head of the malleus must be severed so that the cholesteatoma can be removed successfully.

Painstaking inspection of this area is necessary, and must be repeated several times before it can be judged that the lesions have been totally cured. Such inspection, using mirrors if need be, must always include a systematic checking of the whole of the lower edge of the attic wall and of any pathological notch. Here the inspection is carried out 'blind', using a hook or a spatula in contact with the bony edge, through the attic and through the tympanic cavity. Some of the present authors use a diamond burr to regularize the edge and thus eliminate any remnants of skin that might be adhering to it. It may also be advisable to clean the area with small cotton-wool swabs.

Cholesteatoma Located in the Eustachian Tube

Some of these cholesteatomas may be impossible to treat by surgical means, and a closed-technique operation cannot be used. Others may be removed completely by enlarging the ostium by drilling away the superolateral wall, in order to avoid any risk of damaging the internal carotid.

Cholesteatoma Located in the Windows

Cholesteatomas located here must always be dealt with at the end of the operation, in order to minimize the consequences, which are always serious, of damage to the labyrinth. it is relatively easy to detach the skin from the footplate when the superstructure of the stapes is absent. These manoeuvres are carried out with great care, using a fine suction tip and hooks. The manoeuvres are of the same type as those used to detach squamous epithelium from the secondary tympanic membrane of the round window.

Removal may be much more difficult, however, if the superstructure of the stapes is covered by squamous epithelium. Dissection will proceed from behind forwards along the tendon because of the stapediovestibular joint, the hinge of which is essentially posterior. Patience and care are very necessary. In some cases it is better to leave rather than run the risk of damaging the labyrinth, in the knowledge that, at the routine second-look stage, it may be easier to remove a residual pearl. Cholesteatomas, in these locations, always difficult to eradicate, are to be compared with cholesteatomas, and especially squamous epithelium, on the ossicles. Even if the ossicular chain is intact und mobile, complete eradication can only be achieved by sacrificing it. Likewise, the tympanic membrane must be sacrificed in cases where there is a cholesteatoma on its medial surface.

Fistulae, closed by a cholesteatoma matrix, of the lateral semicircular canal are similar. They too are to be dealt with at the end of the operation in order to minimize, yet again, the consequences of damage to the labyrinth. The surgeon must be extremely careful when dissecting a matrix from the lateral semicircular canal, since the presence of a fistula must always be suspected. Every effort must be made to detect it, after removal of the squamous epithelium in this area by suction, by palpating the matrix with a blunt probe to search for any zone which gives under pressure, and by looking for any sign that movements of the stapes are passed on the fistula. Once the fistula has been identified, great care must be taken to dissect the matrix while preserving the underlying fibrous tissue. If removal seems difficult, it is advisable to leave the skin over the fistula and remove it as a pearl during the second-look stage.

Quite apart from these locations which we have dealt with in great detail, the difficulty encountered in some cases of diffuse squamous epithelialization of the medial wall of the tympanic cavity must be stressed. The presence of such squamous epithelium often requires the sacrifice, to a greater or lesser extent, of the underlying mucosa from which it cannot be detached [159]. In such cases, some of the present authors use sheets of silastic [38] to line the medial wall of the middle ear from the opening of the Eustachian tube as far as the antrum. The aim of interposing this material is, as we have seen, to aid the regeneration of the mucosa by counteracting the growth of fibrous tissue. The present authors use thick silastic if they are simply going to close the tympanic cavity during this first stage, or thin silastic which can be nicked or pierced if the ossicular chain is to be repaired simultaneously. In any event, the sheets of silastic will be removed during the second-look stage. Other authors use gelfilm because it is resorbable.

Reconstruction of the Bony Annulus

Erosion of the attic wall and of the posterosuperior angle is very common in cases of chronic otitis media with cholesteatoma. In this connection, let us stress the absolute necessity to reconstruct the missing part in order to avoid, above all, the recurrence of a retraction pocket, a true precursor of cholesteatoma and secondarily, to ensure support for the new tympanic membrane. A nonresorbable material which is both stable and in harmony with the other walls of the annulus and canal should be used. The reconstruction must only be embarked upon after a careful search has revealed no remnants of skin. These may often be found in the pathological notch. The materials mainly used are bone and cartilage.

Reconstruction of the Attic Wall with a Fragment of Bone

The bone graft is taken from the mastoid cortex. Its size will depend on the quantity of lost bone to be replaced. It must be thick enough to produce a smooth contour. It is shaped to be the desired degree of concavity using a medium-sized eight-toothed burr. The surrounding area must be thinned in such a way that the bone graft will fit

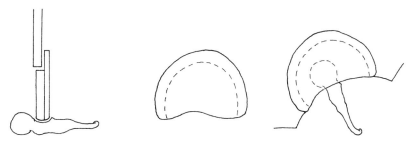

Fig. 75. Repair of attic wall using bone fragment.

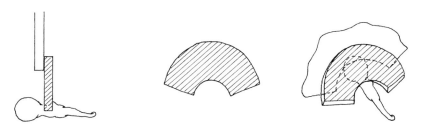

Fig. 76. Repair of attic wall with fragment of cartilage from concha.

into the gap, with a slight relief to stop it from tipping into the attic. It may be advisable to drill away the edges of the eroded area in order to ensure a better fit. The use of a little bone dust with fibrin glue to seal the repair is useful in some cases (fig. 75).

Reconstruction of the Attic Wall with a
Fragment of Cartilage

The cartilage is taken either from a part of the concha where it already has the desired concavity or from the tragus. Some of the present authors use preserved nasal septum. The size will depend on the quantity of lost bone to be replaced. The fragment is held in place inferiorly by a notch made in its inferior edge, allowing it to rest on the neck of the malleus. Superiorly, for some of the present authors, the edge or the cartilage, greatly thinned, is placed on the edge of the gap,

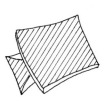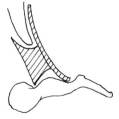

Fig. 77. Repair of attic wall with fragment of preserved nasal septum.

overlapping slightly. For others, the cartilage is held in place at the edge by means of a U-shaped notch [53], the free edge of the bony gap being inserted into the U (fig. 76, 77). A simple and effective technique is to use a piece of cartilage from the tragus, including its thin posterior perichondrium, and with its anterior surface thinned using a knife. This piece of cartilage and perichondrium is quite sufficient to cover the attic wall and the eroded area, beyond which it spreads anteriorly, posteriorly and medially. Whatever the procedure, fibrin glue is very useful to stabilize the reconstruction.

Procedures for Reconstruction of the
Tympanic Membrane and the Ossicular Chain

Any closed-technique operation in a case of chronic otitis media with cholesteatoma is bound to involve closure of the tympanic cavity by a new tympanic membrane, possibly accompanied by the reconstruction of the ossicular chain if the state of the mucosa will permit it. We have decided not to go into too much detail on this subject which does not appear to be confined to cases of chronic otitis media with cholesteatoma.

Materials for Reconstruction of the Tympanic Membrane. Different authors prefer different materials: fascia, perichondrium, or tympanic homograft. These latter two are preferred by some of the present authors because of their texture which makes them possibly more likely than fascia to resist the appearance of retraction pockets.

Materials for Reconstruction of Ossicular Chain. Autografts may be invaded by cholesteatoma. Homografts must be used or prostheses

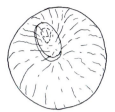

Fig. 78. Diagram of reconstruction of ossicular chain seen through transparent fascia membrane.

(malleus piston, TORP, PORP or ceramic). For some of the present authors, ossicles, when used, must present a transverse carrying surface more likely to resist a retraction pocket, whether it is a type II (complete stapes) or type III (footplate only) operation (fig. 78). The advantage of the total tympano-ossicular homograft is that it obliterates the attic in a manner which is both anatomical and physiological, thus making the appearance of a retraction pocket less likely. As for the new prostheses, the passage of time seems to be disqualifying them in turn.

Variations of the Closed Technique

Feldmann [67, 68] has described a technique which consists of removing the posterosuperior wall of the bony canal temporarily in order to make it easier to remove the lesions from the antro-atticomastoid cavity, the facial recess and the area around the windows. He removes the canal with a special saw which cuts the edges of the bony canal in the shape of a U. Then, after the lesions have been removed, he replaces the posterosuperior wall of the bony canal. It may also be noted that Wullstein [259] has described a similar technique which is only applicable to the attic wall.

Routine Second Look in Closed-Technique Operations

This second step is, for the present authors, routine in all cases of cholesteatoma and in cases of squamous epithelial change when this is widespread. This is, indeed, our only reason for always employing a closed technique – the routine second look. We carry out this second-look operation between 12 and 18 months after the first operation. This seems to us to be a reasonable period, since it gives the mucosa time to recover its normal appearance and also because, when there is a residual cholesteatoma, it is usually no bigger than a pearl. Other surgeons, including Portmann, Marquet and Jansen, do not seem to effect a routine second look.

The aim is threefold:

(1) To search for a residual cholesteatoma. Although it is often encapsulated, there are cases in which its diffuse nature and uncertain limits mean that the choice must be made between a second closed-technique operation to be followed by a third look of which the patient has received notice, or rather a transformation into an open-technique tympanoplasty.

(2) To verify whether certain signs, from which true recurrence of cholesteatoma linked to persistent Eustachian tube malfunction might be predicted, are present. Such signs include retraction pockets or certain inflammatory lesions of the mucosa. If these are found to be present, it may be necessary to supplement ventilation through the Eustachian tube by means of ventilation tube inserted through the tympanic membrane.

(3) To improve hearing further by reconstructing the ossicular chain when this was not done during the first operation, either deliberately or because of problems with the mucosa. If reconstruction was attempted without success during the first operation, a second attempt may be made to improve hearing.

We shall limit our description to those aspects which are specific to these second-look operations. Technically, the operation must be extremely thorough, and at the same time very careful, in order not to prejudice any functional improvement already achieved. This implies an exploration of all the middle ear cavities, which implies in our opinion the choice of a posterior approach. The course of the operation will be determined by the operative record from the first operation, which will include in particular a note of the areas where the removal of the cholesteatoma did not seem satisfactory.

It is usual to find an antro-atticomastoid cavity which is considerably smaller than the operative record would have suggested. This is because there is often a true regeneration of the mastoid cortex. The state of the mucosa in this cavity sometimes suggests immediately whether a cholesteatoma is present or not. If the mucosa is smooth, aerated and luminous, this suggests a healthy ear. If, on the other hand, the mucosa is thick, more or less obliterating the mastoid cavity with obvious fibrous septa, cholesterol granuloma type lesions or glue, this suggests the presence of a cholesteatoma which often appears as soon as the mucosa is incised. It then becomes apparent that this was the matrix of the retraction pocket.

Exploration of the tympanic cavity itself must, of course, take into account the data in the operative record from the previous operation, but as a general rule the residual cholesteatoma is to be looked for in certain selective areas: the epitympanum, the facial recess, the posterior part of the mesotympanum, around the windows and the hypotympanum.

These residual cholesteatomas are generally in the form of a pearl and, in any event, encapsulated, which means that their removal is satisfactory. They may however be diffuse, extending to several areas. It is obviously never possible in such cases to be sure that the removal has been complete. In these cases there is a choice between a second closed-technique operation, involving a third look of which the patient must be informed, and an open-technique tympanoplasty or even a radical mastoidectomy. Experience has shown that cavities obtained in this way after a first closed-technique operation are perfectly stable.

During the second-look operation, if a sheet of silastic has been inserted, it is now removed, and the mucosa often has a surprisingly healthy appearance. The reconstructed columella has every chance of being a success in such cases since, on the one hand, the tympanic membrane is in its final postition and, on the other, the mucosa is healthy. The problem of reconstruction is here essentially a mechanical one.

Technique for Removal of Cholesteatomas of the Middle Ear Extending to the Petrous Bone

Whatever the type of pneumatization of the petrous bone, cholesteatoma may spread from the middle ear into the petrous bone in three main directions. Superiorly, the cholesteatoma may pass in front of the posterior labyrinth, and above the geniculate ganglion, or else behind the posterior labyrinth; in both cases, it may spread above the internal auditory canal and the first portion of the facial nerve. The cholesteatoma may also extend inferiorly below the labyrinth, spreading either generally backwards or generally forwards within the infralabyrinthine cell tracts. The spread of the cholesteatoma may or may not destroy cochlear function, sometimes despite the presence of a fistula, or even of widespread amputation of the labyrinth. The cholesteatoma is of course in a state of unstable balance with the labyrinthine fluids. Its removal often causes deafness.

Posterior and Superior Extension

An extension behind the labyrinth can be dealt with by the otological approach unless it has spread beyond the labyrinth either medially or superiorly. The choice of approach will depend on whether hearing has been preserved or destroyed.

If Hearing Has Been Preserved
The surgeon, while conscious of the risk of failure, should attempt to preserve hearing. The otological route should be combined, in the same operation, with a middle fossa approach, which will follow it.

Otological Route. The ideal technique is the closed technique, since the second-look operation is carried out with healthy mucosa. A cholesteatoma surrounding the posterior and superior semicircular canal must also be followed as far as possible. Extra visiblity can probably be gained by collapsing the lateral sinus. At the end of this step, it is useful to drill the tegmen with a diamond burr in order to identify exactly the point where drilling will start through the middle fossa approach.

Middle Fossa Approach. The usual middle fossa approach is made. Care must be taken to detach the cholesteatoma progressively from the dura mater – the most difficult part of the operation. The cholesteatoma is then dissected, after the internal auditory meatus has been identified if the size of the cholesteatoma seems to endanger the facial nerve. It is then possible to remove the whole of the cholesteatoma, using the two approaches. Only a cholesteatoma medial to the posterior semicircular canal is difficult to get at. At the end of the operation, the tegmen is reconstructed, using part of the original section of bone. Only when the dura mater is breached will it need to be repaired with a large sheet of fascia.

If Hearing Has Been Destroyed

A translabyrinthine approach is possible and sufficient if the cholesteatoma has not spread beyond the first portion of the facial nerve. It is however insufficient otherwise, and a middle fossa approach is then necessary. The patient must therefore be prepared as in the previous case, for both an otological and a middle fossa approach. The closed technique is by far the best method. If it is impossible, in the case of a CSF fistula, only Rambo's or Fisch's ear exclusion technique can be used.

Translabyrinthine Approach. This is opened as required after the 3rd portion and the genu of the facial nerve have been identified as so to determine how far it is possible to drill. The posterior labyrinth is drilled out and the cholesteatoma is followed as far as the internal auditory meatus and sometimes as far as the pontocerebellar angle. In this latter case it is essential to make a perfect seal by obliterating with abdominal fat. The attic and the posterior tympanotomy must be blocked with fibroperiosteal tissue. Some surgeons may think it more prudent to use Rambo's technique.

Supralabyrinthine Extension

The extension follows the anterior supralabyrinthine cell tract and turns in front of the superior semicircular canal, above the 2nd portion of the facial nerve, to develop medially to the superior semicircular canal and the vestibule, in contact with the 1st portion of the facial nerve, the internal auditory meatus and the cochlea (fig. 79). Whether the hearing has been preserved or destroyed, only a middle fossa approach can give a clear view of the first two portions of the facial nerve, and of the internal auditory meatus up to the point where the nerve passes under the lateral semicircular canal. The middle fossa approach must be combined with the otological route.

Otological Route. The ideal otological route is the closed technique, but an open technique, with or without obliteration, may be used provided there is no breach of the meninges. In such a case, Rambo's technique would be the wisest.

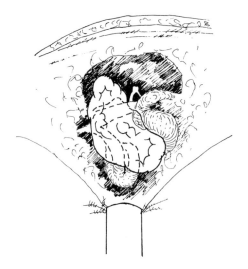

Fig. 79. Cholesteatoma spread from the attic (on the right side) by the anterior supralabyrinthine cell tract to extend above the 2nd and 1st portions of the facial nerve
medially to the denuded vestibule and the skeletonized superior semicircular canal.
Middle fossa approach – hearing preserved.

Middle Fossa Approach. A cholesteatoma located in the middle ear
may be dissected by either the open or the closed technique. Once it
has been removed, a diamond burr is used to mark on the tegmen the
starting-point from which the lesions will be followed by the middle
fossa route. The cholesteatoma matrix should be dissected progressively along with the dura mater. This dissection is difficult. After the
geniculate ganglion and possibly the internal auditory meatus have
been identified, the matrix is lifted, very delicately, from its zone of
bone erosion, since the cochlea and vestibule or canals are very often
closed only by their endosteum. The tegmen must be reconstructed,
and a large graft of fascia is necessary if the dura has been opened.

Infralabyrinthine Extension

Such an extension may be predominantly posterior, inserting itself
between the jugular bulb below, the ampulla of the posterior semicir-

cular canal above and the facial nerve laterally and reaching medially towards the inferior surface of the internal auditory meatus. Or, on the other hand, it may spread forwards, along the internal carotid, or medially, basically underneath the labyrinth. The labyrinth is of course often involved, and there may be many fistulae on its inferior surface if the cholesteatoma reaches a certain volume. Sometimes destruction has gone so far that the bony labyrinth almost appears to be suspended after the cholesteatoma has been removed. Depending on the extent and the location of the lesions, an otological route, combined with an approach between the facial nerve and the sigmoid sinus, or rerouting of the facial nerve, are required.

Otological Aproach Combined with Approach Between Facial Nerve and Sigmoid Sinus and Below the Labyrinth. It is possible, using either a closed or an open technique, to follow the cholesteatoma medially to the facial nerve by opening the posterior infralabyrinthine cell tract between the lateral sinus behind and below, the ampullary branch of the posterior semicircular canal above and the facial nerve anteriorly. First, of course, the posterior surface of the facial nerve must be skeletonized and then its inferior surface, while the posterior semicircular canal and the sinuous route of the sigmoid sinus must be identified. The greatest difficulty is of course in identifying the posterior semicircular canal, especially if the bone is eburnated. It is thus possible to move forward again into the tympanic cavity and dissect a cholesteatoma with a volume of 1 cm^3 located medial to the facial nerve. This technique can be used in conjunction with a closed technique operation, and if so, silastic may be left in the approach route and in the posterior tympanotomy, so that they can be checked during the second look. It is also possible in conjunction with an open technique. When this is accompanied by an obliteration, it may be necessary to obliterate this zone where the cholesteatoma would otherwise spread again.

Rerouting of the Facial Nerve. If the extension is of any size, it is essential to reroute the 3rd and 2nd portions of the facial nerve, using the technique which Fisch has described. A large supra-, post- and retroauricular curved incision is made, and the skin, muscle and periosteal flap is folded over anteriorly as in a translabyrinthine approach. The cartilaginous canal is severed level with the concha, which is sutured by stitches which retract the skin outwards (fig. 80). The facial

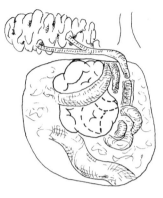

Fig. 80. Large cholesteatoma in the left middle ear, extending below the labyrinth, destroying the cochlea and exposing the internal carotid over its posterior, medial and anterior surfaces. Transcochleovestibular route, with rerouting of the 2nd and 3rd portions of the facial nerve.

nerve is identified as in a parotidectomy and its bifurcation is freed slightly. A large cavity is then opened after the bony canal skin and the tympanic membrane have been removed. A large antro-atticomastoidectomy, removing as much as possible of the bony canal makes it possible to identify the facial nerve in its 2nd and 3rd portions. The anterior and inferior wall of the bony canal is removed level with the temporomandibular joint so as to uncover the protympanum and the hypotympanum. A groove is made in the foot of the zygoma for the facial nerve. This is then extracted in its sheath and with great care from the stylomastoid foramen to the geniculate ganglion. It is loosely suspended inside the parotid gland.

The whole of the medial surface of the labyrinth is thus cleared, and the lesions may be followed posteriorly between the jugular bulb and the lower part of the lateral sinus, and anteriorly between the ascending portion and the bend of the internal carotid. It is then possible to continue the dissection medial to these vessels. This is the stage at which it may become necessary to sacrifice the labyrinth; access is then only limited superiorly by the internal auditory meatus and the first portion of the facial nerve, both of which must be approached with care. Anteriorly it is possible to open the protympanum anterior to the internal carotid to gain better visibility. It may be possible to continue as far as the middle meningeal artery and the mandibular nerve in the oval foramen. Once the cholesteatoma has been carefully dissected, the operation is completed by an obliteration using fatty tissue.

There is thus a suitable technique for each type of extension of cholesteatoma of the middle ear into the petrous bone. Appropriate tomography must therefore be made routinely before any cholesteatoma is operated on in order to find these extensions. This is because the area to be shaved, the length of the operation, the degree of risk to the facial nerve and especially to the inner ear, all vary considerably from case to case. CAT scanner and MRI must be performed for studying size and extension. The patient must be informed of the size of the lesion and of the subsequent treatment involved. These single-stage operations are definitely preferable to complementary operations which always leave uncertainty over the point of correlation with the previous procedure, and which endanger the facial nerve and the labyrinth to a greater degree during the otological approach.

Indications

It is unanimously agreed in principle that only surgical treatment is suitable for cholesteatoma, except for a few rare contraindications. We shall simply note in passing the medical treatment advocated quite some time ago by McGukin [145] and Verhoeven [247]; it consisted of suction of the cholesteatomatous material from retraction pocket, or through a perforation, using angled suction tips. We shall also mention the work of Kluyskens [121] who insufflates acetylcysteine powder in some cases of attic cholesteatoma. This appears to make their removal, by washing and suction, easier.

Smyth [219] in his treatise on 'Chronic ear disease', goes as far as to compare the risks involved in surgery to those involved in refraining from surgery, and claims that there are more complications as a result of the surgical act than of the causative disease. We do not share this opinion. All cholesteatomas, in our view, should be treated surgically. The choice of modalities to adopt, set out schematically, seems to depend on the disease, the patient, and finally the surgeon. But we wish to point out, before going further, that in our opinion there is no 'best' technique, and we have no intention of embarking on a defense of the closed technique against the open technique or vice versa. In our view, all the various techniques can be equally successful, provided that the indications are correct and the operation is properly carried out.

No surgical treatment, in fact, whether simple or sophisticated, radical or reconstructive, can claim to achieve a permanent cure in every case, since there is always the uncertainty of the pathogenesis of cholesteatoma and especially our inability to master all aspects of Eustachian tube malfunction. Before going on to consider the indications in cases of cholesteatoma of the middle ear, we shall give a brief summary of the various attitudes we have noted, taken either from the literature on the subject or from the completed questionnaires which were returned to us. We have only taken into account statistically significant series of more than 100 cases. This is, unavoidably, a mere outline, and we hope that we are not unduly misrepresenting the ideas of the various authors. Surgeons may be divided into three categories: those who almost always use a closed technique; those who almost always use an open technique, and those who vary their technique to suit the case.

Among those authors who almost invariably use the closed technique, we find, in alphabetical order: Gersdorff [90], Glasscock [94, 95], Jansen [111, 112, 114, 118], Marquet [245], Pech, Sterkers [230], Strauss and Vergnon [233]. It is interesting to note that these authors adopt different attitudes towards the principle of the second-look operation. Jansen, for example, never carries out second-look surgery, but keeps the ear under regular observation and, apparently, carries out a transcutaneous antroscopy using a Storz's endoscope. Sheehy [202, 203, 208, 209, 213] and Strauss carry out the second-look operation in 70% of their cases and Gersdorff in 45%. Marquet, finally, divides his patients into three categories – second look, no second look, and borderline. It is to be noted that these authors sometimes carry out a radical mastoidectomy. Wullstein [259], lastly, sticks to the osteoplastic epitympanotomy, a variation on the closed technique; she will only occasionally carry out a second look.

Some authors, on the other hand, only use the open technique either with management of the tympanic cavity (Cotin, for example, carries out a second-look operation whenever possible, 2 years after the operation), or with management of the posterior cavity. Some of these surgeons use a Palva's flap – Montandon [147], Palmgren [153] and Palva [156, 157, 160]. Pfaltz [163, 164] reconstructs the posterior canal wall using cartilage and lyophilized dura mater.

In fact, most authors vary their technique to suit the individual case, but they nonetheless display a preference for one technique or the other: Bremond [24], Portmann [170], Zini [261, 262], for example, seem to have a marked preference for the closed technique. Ansart, Bluestone, De Paepe, Fleury [75], Fombeur [80], and Klein and Sakai [192], on the other hand, seem more inclined to use an open technique. Fisch [72], Limbour, Martin [143], Plester [167], Smyth [221–223] and Tos [237, 239, 242] form a third group of surgeons who seem to use the open and closed techniques in statistically equal proportions. Obliteration of the posterior cavity is favoured by some authors [208, 243].

Whatever the extent to which they prefer one technique or the other, most of these authors seem to include a more or less planned second look. This is obviously more frequent in the case of those who use a closed technique more especially. The second look seems to be routine for Bremond, Fisch, Smyth and Zini, while it is carried out in half of their cases by Sheehy, Ansart and Fombeur. But even authors who prefer an open technique are concerned to have a second look, either for functional or for anatomical reasons – Fisch, Smyth and Palmgren are examples. Some authors, on the other hand, never have a second look, on principle – Martin and Tos, for example.

In the choice of technique for operating on children, two types of surgeons may be distinguished: some adopt exactly the same attitude as they do for adults – this is the case for Bluestone [21], De Paepe, Jansen [116, 117], Sanna [195], Sakai [192], Sheehy [201, 207], Smyth [220], and Tos [241]; the others adopt a different attitude – Andrieu-Guitrancourt [10], for example, uses open technique predominantly and states that his results from a functional point of view, are better than those obtained from a closed technique. Austin [14] prefers to use a closed technique and, if he is forced to use an open technique, he immediately reconstructs the bony canal, using cartilage. This, we think, is a fair summary of the opinions of the authors who were kind enough to reply to us, although we are well aware that it is, unavoidably, only an outline. Before going on to describe our own attitude to chronic otitis media with cholesteatoma, we wish to give an account of the approach we adopt towards such precursors of cholesteatoma as epidermosis and retraction pockets.

Precursors of Cholesteatoma

Epidermosis

In the chapter on pathological anatomy, we have described these as anarchical migrations of skin in the form of a stream of sheet. They extend either from the edges of a perforation, over the medial surface of the tympanic membrane or, via the chorda tympani, down the long process of the incus even as far as the stapes, its tendon and the surrounding areas, or from a retracted umbo, touching the promontory in such a way as to guide a sheet of skin which will go on to invade the whole floor of the tympanic cavity.

It may be said that these epidermosis illustrate the direct migration theory. Whatever their extent and however well-defined their limits, it must be stressed at once that they must be treated by surgery, since they may always lead to a true cholesteatoma. The surgeon must constantly be on the lookout for them even when performing the simplest of tympanoplasties. In this connection it is essential, in our view, to remind the reader that any perforation must be meticulously examined both before and during surgery in order to judge the extent to which the epidermis has gone beyond the edges of the perforation and has extended to the medial surface of the tympanic membrane.

Even a single residual epidermic cell could be the starting-point for an iatrogenic cholesteatoma. This examination may be carried out using a Zini or Buckingham mirror or Storz's cold light otoscope, looking both towards the medial surface of the tympanic membrane and towards the facial recess and the hypotympanum. The preoperative and operative examination thus enables two main aspects of these epidermosis to be distinguished: (a) *Epidermosis with clear-cut edges:* these may be completely dissected during the preparation of the graft bed. Their removal involves the sacrifice of part of the tympanic membrane. (b) *Diffuse invasive epidermosis:* their edges are ill-defined, and they are often located on the promontory or in the incudostapedial area, from which they may extend into the facial recess and even the sinus tympani. In these cases, in order to control them, it is necessary to perform a closed-technique tympanoplasty in the manner we have described, with a posterior tympanotomy.

Retraction Pockets

Retraction pockets are found especially in children, and every effort must be made to prevent them from developing into true cholesteatomas. They are characterized by four essential factors on which the indication for surgery depends: (1) whether or not they are fixed; (2) their extent; (3) whether there is accumulation of squamous debris or a self-cleansing pocket, and (4) the degree of infection.

Generally speaking, fixed, extensive desquamating and infected retraction pockets require surgical treatment, the details of which will depend on the location: An *attic retraction pocket* requires a closed-technique tympanoplasty with a posterior tympanotomy, since it is difficult to predict with certainty how far it extends. The attic wall must always be reconstructed as it is always partially eroded. A *posterosuperior retraction pocket,* when it can be circled, may be dealt with by surgical strengthening of the tympanic membrane using perichondrium or cartilage thinned so as to prevent any recurrence. A *posterior retraction pocket,* adherent to the retrotympanum, requires a closed-technique tympanoplasty with a posterior tympanotomy. If the removal does not appear entirely satisfactory, a second look is necessary. A *movable, limited, nondesquamating retraction pocket* which is not infected, on the other hand – a type frequently observed in children – should be inspected regularly and receive medial treatment: adenoidectomy, rhinosinusal treatment, crenotherapy, beta-therapy in certain cases, transtympanic aeration, Eustachian tube exercises. In some cases, surgical reinforcement of the tympanic membrane may be envisaged.

Cholesteatomas Without Complications in Adults

Although some surgeons have taken a dogmatic view which seems excessive to us, the indications depend above all on: the characteristics of the mastoid on one hand (in general terms, it may be pneumatized, sclerotic or eburnated); the characteristics of the cholesteatoma on the other hand (in general terms, it may be encapsulated, in a hernial sac, diffuse or ramifying). Inspection of the mastoid is indeed, in our view, an essential parameter, since on it will depend the size of the mastoid cavity. We have already seen that one of the preconditions for a mastoid cavity which will be simple to follow up is the total removal of the mastoid cells. If the mastoid is widely pneumatized, the result will be a very large cavity which, however it is managed, may be the seat of more or less permanent infection, making the patient's life uncomfortable. If the cells removal has been incomplete, moreover, the mucosa of these remaining cells, being no longer aerated, may give rise to lesions of the cholesterol granuloma type, which may in turn be a source of otorrhoea. Cholesteatomas developing in pneumatized mastoids are to be found particularly in children, and this will of course influence the indications for treatment. In adults, however, pneumatization of the mastoid is generally less pronounced.

Pneumatized Mastoid

In view of the above, a highly pneumatized mastoid, whatever the type or size of the cholesteatoma, requires in our view a two-stage closed technique with a systematic second look, which will be carried out between 12 and 18 months after the operation, and thus ensure that no undesirable developments have occurred. We thus avoid the disadvantages of an open technique, which would leave an enormous mastoid cavity, requiring a large and unattractive conchoplasty. Obliteration would be both inadequate and potentially dangerous because of the risk of epidermal inclusion and exclusion of the cell tracts, which may develop cholesterol granuloma-type lesions. With long experience it is possible to judge how unstable these large cavities are, cavities which do not protect the patient from complications linked to a recurrence of the cholesteatoma, such as a fistula of the lateral semicircular canal, or intracranial complications [73, 240].

Sclerotic or Eburnated Mastoid

The compact nature of the bone forms a natural defence barrier, and the small size of the cavity removes many of the objections to the open technique in these cases.

When the Open Technique Is Indicated. First, there are the cases where technical problems are caused by certain anatomical peculiarities such as a low dura or a forward sinus. This sort of problem seems to be easier to handle when using an open technique. Malfunction of the Eustachian tube must also be taken into account, and will tend to indicate an open technique. This is because the risk of retraction pocket, which might be present in such cases if a closed technique were used, disappears when the open technique is adopted, since, by definition, there is no bony canal. It may also be expected that the reduced volume of the tympanic cavity, reconstructed as part of an open technique, will be better adapted to ventilation via the Eustachian tube. This is true in cases of chronic otitis media with cholesteatoma in patients with a cleft palate and its sequelae, a submucous cleft of the soft palate of a bifid uvula. Obliteration of the mastoid cavity using a Palva flap in these open-technique tympanoplasties ensures stability by the quality of the connective tissue. On the other hand, however, the risk of inclusion of epidermis under the flap means, in our view, that this technique is only indicated in cases where the cholesteatoma has not invaded the mastoid cavity.

When the Closed Technique Is Indicated. Discovery during surgery of a greater number of pneumatized cells than had been expected, involving the opening of a larger cavity, may constitute one indication. Another case might be the discovery of an extensive cholesteatoma where the extension is lamellar and extensive bone-work again becomes necessary – a closed technique would thus be preferable.

We have just seen the main arguments in favour of one technique or the other, but the choice between them may also be seen in terms of other parameters. Some of these relate to the patient: his agreement to undergo a second stage of surgery, the possibility of regular long-term follow-up and inspection, which is in fact necessary whichever technique is chosen, and personal factors such as life-style, hygiene, profession, past history and financial factors. Others relate to the disease, although in fact accompanying infectious pathology does not modify the criteria of choice mentioned above. Others, finally, relate to the state of the inner ear; a poor cochlear reserve in the operated ear generally tends to indicate an open technique, possibly with obliteration. In such cases the surgeon cannot hope to attempt to improve hearing; with a poor cochlear reserve in the opposite ear, the surgeon must be extremely careful, and therefore use the technique which, for him, will involve the least risk to this ear, which must be considered as a single ear.

To conclude this section, we should like to say that we are well aware that our indications in the treatment of cholesteatoma in adults are inevitably only an outline. The various criteria can only point in the general direction, which may obviously be modified in the light of operative findings. To sum up, the best technique is the technique which in the short term allows the complete eradication of the cholesteatoma and will ensure that the anatomical and functional results will be permanent in the future.

Indications Depending on Age

Children

A certain number of factors are peculiar to children: the fact that mastoids in which the cholesteatoma develops are commonly pneumatized, the fact that the cholesteatomas are often extensive and even finger-like, the special nature of the cholesteatoma's potential for development, the fact that most cholesteatomas stem from an obvious dysfunction of the Eustachian tube, the immunological instability which is characteristic of children, and, finally, the fact that disorders of bone growth are sometimes observed in the middle ear after an open technique.

As a consequence of what we have said on the subject of pneumatization of the mastoid, we often have an a priori preference for the closed technique. This is all the more true because it is particularly easy to perform on children, and especially worthwhile because the likelihood that hearing will be improved is much greater at this age. It also avoids any restrictions on the pleasures of bathing. However, the fact that the cholesteatomas are often extensive, with a finger-like form, the special nature of their potential for development, and the immunological instability characteristic of children, all tend to cast doubt on the permanent nature of the result of the operation, since recurrence of infection is so common. In the light of this, the surgeon may modify the indication for a closed technique and adopt rather an open-technique tympanoplasty, with the intention of reconstucting the ear at a later date, from anatomical, and possibly even a functional, point of view. If a closed technique has been decided upon, the second-look operation is more necessary than ever, and in the view of some of the present authors, should be carried out earlier, given the progressive nature of the residual cholesteatoma.

Dysfunction of the Eustachian tube, finally, may require transtympanic aeration as part of the follow-up to the operation. It may also mean, if a retraction pocket is found during the second look, that a closed technique should be transformed into an open technique, with obliteration, if necessary, of the mastoid cavity. The problems raised by cholesteatoma in children are a matter of some controversy, as can be seen from the widely varying therapeutic attitudes found in the literature on the subject. Mauer, Jansen and Sheehy, for example, use the closed technique routinely, drawing no distinction between children and adults, while Palmgren [153], on the other hand, only uses the open technique.

Old People

The general conditions tend to indicate the use of an open technique, whether it be a tympanoplasty or even a radical mastoidectomy, and this is all the more true in that local conditions are also favourable, the mastoid very often being sclerotic. It is moreover obvious that repeated surgery is to be avoided.

Indications Depending on Other Illnesses

Diabetics

In general the most characteristic factor is the fact that the healing time is long. The choice of technique appears to be of little importance. However, in the view of one of the present authors, the best results are obtained by using an open technique, with a Palva flap obliteration. As a general rule, the surgeon must choose the type of operation which will give an immediate and permanent result, in order to avoid further surgery.

Patients Suffering from Bronchiectasis

Indications for treatment are governed by the poor quality of the mucosa of the airways and upper digestive tracts, often associated with immobility of the cilia (Kartagener's, Mounier-Kühn's and Garderes' syndromes). Secondly, cholesteatomas in such patients have rather special characteristics: they are in fact more often epidermal plugs than true cholesteatomas. They tend to develop into the form of a dilated gourd and even towards spontaneous excavation. Surgery is rarely indicated, treatment usually being confined to repeated suction.

Particular Cases

Development of Cholesteatoma Beneath a Postoperative
Stenosis of the External Auditory Meatus

Such a cholesteatoma may be detected on the occurrence of a complication. An open-technique tympanoplasty will obviously be used to deal with both the cholesteatoma and the stenosis at the same time.

Cholesteatoma in a Single Ear

We share the opinion of those authors, including Aboulker et al. [1, 2], for whom the rule that a cholesteatoma must receive surgical treatment is not to be waived because the cholesteatoma is in the patient's only functional ear. We would even go as far as to advocate that the surgery be performed as soon as possible since, at any rate in theory, the operation is likely to be less difficult from a technical point of view. This view is not however shared by all authors. We only adopt a 'wait and see' attitude in a case where there is a retraction pocket conforming to the criteria we have already laid down (not extensive, without squamous debris and not infected). Once it has been decided to operate, the surgeon will choose the technique which puts the patient in the least risk. In any event, the patient must be warned that his deafness may become more pronounced and that he may have to resort to the use of a hearing aid.

Cholesteatoma with Fistula of the Lateral Semicircular Canal in a Single Ear

Although, in general, a cholesteatoma matrix over a fistula may be dissected when there is underlying connective tissue, it is out of the question to envisage any surgical manoeuvre when it is in the patient's only functional ear. An open technique therefore must be performed.

Cholesteatoma in a Totally Deaf Ear

If the ear has not been operated on previously: In principle, we tend to perform an open-technique tympanoplasty, but in fact the choice of a technique depends, here again, on the characteristics of the mastoid and of the cholesteatoma, and on individual factors such as the patient's profession or leisure activities.

If the ear has been operated on previously: (a) If the previous operation used an open technique, only an open technique can of course be used now, but the cavity should be reshaped and managed by obliteration or meatoconchoplasty, or using both combined. In some cases a complete exclusion using Rambo's technique may be necessary [147]. (b) If the previous operation used a closed technique, it is often but not invariably necessary to change this closed technique into an open technique.

Indications for the Treatment of Residual Cholesteatomas

The expression 'residual cholesteatoma' [210, 212, 214, 217, 218] is used to describe any epidermal inclusion left in the cavities of the middle ear. In most cases, this in not intended by the surgeon, and is a result of inadequate surgery. But in certain cases the epidermis is left in place intentionally – on stapes for example. Rather than risk a vestibular complication, the surgeon postpones the removal until a planned second stage when, in theory at least, it will have taken the form of an easily-removed pearl. These residual cholesteatomas are usually encapsulated in the form of a pearl or a cyst. When they are diffuse, it is very difficult to be certain that their eradication has been complete. There are two types of case, depending on whether the residual cholesteatoma has developed on an open-technique or a closed-technique tympanoplasty.

Residual Cholesteatoma Which Has Developed on an Open Technique Tympanoplasty

This type of cholesteatoma may be discovered during a routinely planned operation, or indeed during an operation whose aim is to improve hearing which was insufficiently improved during a first operation.

Residual cholesteatoma which has developed in the tympanic cavity: If encapsulated, it is easy to remove, if, on the other hand, it is diffuse, taking the form of a trickle or drop of candlewax, then it is likely to be more difficult to remove. If the removal seems to have been satisfactory, the tympanic cavity may be closed again. If not, a radical mastoidectomy may be necessary. In this case the Eustachian tube must be blocked if possible.

Cholesteatoma which has developed on an obliteration tympanoplasty: If this residual cholesteatoma is encapsulated, the muscle flap may be preserved. If not, it must be sacrificed.

Residual Cholesteatoma Discovered During Closed-Technique Surgery

Let us state again that, for us, such residual cholesteatomas in closed-technique surgery will be discovered during the systematically planned second stage operation between a year and 18 months after the first operation. All will depend on the appearances of this cholesteatoma: (1) If it is encapsulated, it is generally very easy to remove – this is the case for 'pearls' and 'cysts'. If the cholesteatoma is encapsulated but much more extensive it may be necessary to sacrifice the tympanic membrane, and if there is the slightest doubt as to whether the cholesteatoma has been completely removed, a third stage operation must be performed – the patient having obviously been warned of such an eventuality. (2) If the cholesteatoma is diffuse, the indication is more problematical. It is to be noted that such an aspect is rarely found in the antrum or the mastoid, but is essentially confined to the tympanic cavity (the posterior half of the tympanic cavity and the hypotympanum) and in the attic. A radical mastoidectomy with blocking of the Eustachian tube may be required.

Indications for Treatment of Retraction Pocket

A retraction pocket in the months or years following the treatment of chronic otitis media with cholesteatoma by two-stage closed-technique surgery would appear to be proof of persistent tubal dysfunction. Treatment of this true recurrence of cholesteatoma depends on its size. If it is small, either ventilation of the tympanic cavity may be improved by a trans-tympanic aeration tube, or the tympanic membrane may be reinforced and the dimensions of the annulus reduced by surgery as described above. If it is larger, a second operation is required, and this may reveal the existence of a true cholesteatoma. The persistent tubal dysfunction, which makes it theoretically impossible to attempt closed-technique tympanolasty again, must be taken into account. It will therefore be necessary to perform an open-technique tympanoplasty with or without a Palva's flap. This type of secondarily open tympanoplasty gives stable cavities; the net result is as if the mastoid bone had reacted in such a way as to ensure an improved trophicity of the flap or of its covering skin, the remaining elements of the tympanic membrane being quite stable and making for optimum efficiency of the functional management of the tympanic cavity. In conclusion, these true recurrences are examples of the final challenge – that of disorder function of the Eustachian tube, many factors of which are still unknown.

Results

Report on the Present Author's Results

We have sought to improve the statistical value of our results by combining our different series. A few minor variations will become apparent in the course of our report, particularly concerning open techniques (radical mastoidectomies, open-technique tympanoplasty with management of the tympanic cavity, with or without obliteration of the posterior cavities). The preferences of each individual surgeon are shown in table II. These results have been expressed so as to correspond to the questionnaire which we sent to our colleagues in otology. In particular, it should be noted that the series only includes patients operated upon between 1st January 1974 and 31st December 1978. This series includes 1,856 cases (cholesteatomas and fixed retraction pockets on which the same techniques were used). The results were analysed by computer.

Open Techniques

Radical Mastoidectomies
We performed 175 radical mastoidectomies, but the proportions vary greatly from series to series – from 0/529 to 110/312 cholesteatomas. For two surgeons, the indication for radical mastoidectomy was practically confined to major complications of cholesteatomas of the middle ear. These mastoid cavities are all too often unstable (in 35% of cases).

Open-Technique Tympanoplasty with
Management of the Tympanic Cavity
The combined series includes 374 cases, but the number of open-technique tympanoplasties varies between 8 and 176 in the individual series.

Table II. Cholesteatoma surgery, 1974–1978

	Radical mastoid-ectomy	Open-technique tympanoplasty		Closed-technique tympano-plasty
		with management of the tympanic cavity	with management of the tympanic cavity and obliteration of posterior cavity	
Wayoff	2	176	8	78
Charachon	17	8	196	216
Roulleau	110	24	0	178
Lacher	46	13	2	253
Deguine	0	153	0	376

Results from an Anatomical Point of View

The number of residual perforations, some of them with otor-rhoea, varies between 1.5 and 2% for the two largest series (153 and 176 cases). No revision of the tympanic cavity was carried out. The residual cholesteatomas therefore became apparent through their development behind the graft. They were extremely limited in number in the two largest series (153 and 176 cases), varying between 2.6 and 1.6%. In a considerably smaller series, they were present in 23% of 13 cases. The posterior cavities were found to be unstable much less frequently than in radical mastoidectomies. In the two largest series (153 and 176 cases), wet cavities were observed in 9 and 6.5% of the cases.

Results From a Functional Point of View

These were calculated, as for the whole of our series, by the gap between air conduction 4 months after the operation and bone conduction before the operation, based on the average thresholds at 500, 1,000 and 2,000 Hz.

In one of the largest series (153 cases), the following results were obtained:

39	*intact stapes*			19	*missing crura*		
ABG	AC–BC	< 10 dB	17%	ABG	AC–BC	< 10 dB	20%
ABG	AC–BC	< 20 dB	61%	ABG	AC–BC	< 20 dB	60%

Open-Technique Tympanoplasty with Management of the
Tympanic Cavity and Obliteration of the Posterior Cavities

Our series brings together 206 cases. In actual fact, one surgeon, mainly using Palva's flap, provides a series of 196 cases on his own.

Results From an Anatomical Point of View

Perforation was observed in 1% ot these cases. Seromucous otitis media, however, appeared in 2.5% of the cases over the 5 years during which they were followed up. Revision of the tympanic cavity was only performed in 62% of the 196 cases in the largest series. This made it possible to detect and remove a residual cholesteatoma pearl in 16% of the cases, and to reconstruct the ossicular chain. The flap was not lifted in any of the cases, and only one residual cholesteatoma appeared underneath the flap. Five retraction pockets (2.5% of the cases) appeared however in the flap, involving 3 further operations.

Results From a Functional Point of View

In the series of 196 cases, it was only possible to analyze the results from a functional point of view in 152 cases. This was because a certain number of second-stage operations, which had originally be planned, could not be performed.

83	*intact stapes*			69	*missing crura*		
ABG	AC–BC	<10 dB	30%	ABG	AC–BC	<10 dB	20%
ABG	AC–BC	<20 dB	64%	ABG	AC–BC	<20 dB	48%

Closed Techniques

Our series includes 1,101 cases in which closed techniques were used in the way we have described, i.e. with a posterior tympanotomy which is the only method of eradicating the epidermis completely.

Results From a Anatomical Point of View

Perforations of the tympanic membrane appeared in 4% of the cases overall, ranging from 2 to 5% in individual series. These 4% include both dry perforations (3%) and discharging perforations. The second-look stage was only performed by 4 of us during the period in question, in a total of 63% of the cases, a percentage which varies from

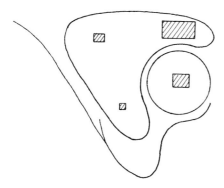

Fig. 81. Location of residual cholesteatomas in closed-technique surgery (550 second looks).

36 to 72% in individual series. The fifth surgeon only began to perform the second look during the fifth year of the period. Residual cholesteatomas were discovered in 44.5% of the cases during the second look. This percentage varies from 12 to 55% in individual series.

The residual cholesteatomas were judged too large or too diffuse, so as to justify abandoning the closed technique in 15 cases out of 533 second-look operations – 2.80%. In 16 cases (3%), it was decided that the closed technique could only still be used if there was a third stage – a second revision – performed 1 or 2 years later, revealing no further lesions. The location of these residual cholesteatomas varies somewhat from one series to another, but they were most common in the attic and the tympanic cavity (fig. 81). The macroscopical appearances of the residual cholesteatomas varied. In 80% of these residual cholesteatomas, there were completely encapsulated pearls; in 1 case out of 8 there were multiple pearls. In 20% of these residual cholesteatomas, the lesions were considerably more severe – either large pearls (8%) or ill-defined masses of epidermis (12%).

Attic	29–55%	average 46%
Tympanic cavity	14–52%	average 30%
Antrum	7–25%	average 17%
Mastoid	2–12%	average 6%

It was possible to compare two of our individual series of statistics in an attempt to assess the difference between the tendency to development in adults and in children. In one series, the percentage of pearls was approximately the same for both adults and children. In the other series, the percentage was 46% for children (19 pearls out of 41 second-look operations) as against 27% for adults (25 pearls out of 93 second-look operations).

Seromucous otitis appeared as a more or less delayed sequela in between 1.6 and 3% of the cases. A transtympanic aeration tube must be inserted in such cases. In the overall series, a retraction pocket appeared in 10% of the cases, generally during the first 3 years of follow-up, and more rarely later. It varied between 8 and 16% of the cases in the individual series. Temporary or permanent insertion of silastic does not appear to be an important factor in preventing these pockets, although one of our individual series shows a difference between closed techniques, with a second look, involving the temporary inclusion of thick silastic (5% after 3 years) and closed techniques, without a second look, only involving thin silastic (13% after 3 years). These retraction pockets were serious enough to warrant further surgery, either, for two surgeons, surgery to reinforce the tympanic membrane in 50% of the cases, or in the other cases and for the other surgeons, to switch to an open technique, with or without obliteration depending on the extent of the pocket and each surgeon's individual preferences.

Results From a Functional Point of View

We have not separated the results according to whether a second-look operation was performed or not, although, in one series, results appeared to be better from a functional point of view when the stapes was destroyed and ossicular chain was reconstructed during the second look:

58 *intact ossicular chain*	*262* *intact stapes*	*195* *missing crura*
ABG AC–BC <10 dB 53%	ABG AC–BC <10 dB 37% (30–45%)	ABG AC–BC <10 dB 26% (26–27%)
ABG AC–BC <20 dB 87%	ABG AC–DB <20 dB 69% (67–71%)	ABG AC–BC <20 dB 60% (41–66%)

Total deafness was noted in 1% of cases. The figures vary between 0 out of 216 cases and 7 out of 376, depending on the series. Slight sensorineural loss of 20 dB or more computed on the average of 4,000 and 8,000 Hz appeared in between 2 and 16% of cases depending on the series.

Comments on the Present Author's Results

Choice of Technique

Our results demonstrate the distinctions made in our indications since, as we have said, we used an open technique in 41% of the cases and a closed technique in 59%. This was our attitude during the period in question, but we have since tended to extend the indications for a closed technique. This is a result of several factors. Closed techniques, by their very nature, eliminate the instability of the cavities, which is in our view the major drawback of the open techniques. In this connection, we have observed that when an open technique is used secondarily, the results are considerably more stable than when an open technique is used from the outset. From a functional point of view, the results obtained by closed-technique surgery appear to be noticeably better than those obtained by open techniques, although the difference is less definite than many authors would have us believe. Although the use of a hearing aid may still be necessary, it is better tolerated and more effective. Taken together, these advantages mean that the patient's life will be more comfortable, and in our view they fully justify the need for a systematic second look.

With children, as is shown in table III, the percentage of open and closed techniques are noticeably different from those in the operations on adults. Out of a total of 1,856 cases, 1,460 were adults and 396 children. A closed technique was used in 55.75% of the operations on adults, and 72.40% of those on children. the difference shows the importance accorded by the present authors to the mastoid factor. In children, the all too frequent instability of the cavity may be explained by the extent of pneumatization of the mastoid, giving rise to a cavity which is too large, and the reactivity of the mucosa, favouring infection.

Open Techniques

Standard Radical Mastoidectomy

Except for two of the present authors, who performed it as a matter of principle, the indication for this operation seems to be confined to major complications and cholesteatomas in elderly patients. These operations have become rare because, in most cases where they were

Table III. Cholesteatoma surgery, 1974–1978

	Children			Adults		
	open technique, n	closed technique		open technique, n	closed technique	
		n	%		n	%
Wayoff	31	20	39.2	155	58	27.2
Charachon	27	53	66	194	163	45.6
Roulleau	33	59	64	101	119	54
Lacher	4	36	90	57	217	79.1
Deguine	14	119	89.4	139	257	64.8
Total	109	287	72.4	646	814	55.7

formerly indicated, it is now possible to perform more elaborate surgery of the tympanic cavity, leading to an open-technique tympanoplasty.

Open-Technique Tympanoplasty

The experience gained from performing closed techniques has led us to apply the same strict rules to dissection and reconstruction in open techniques. Should such a reconstruction be confined to the tympanic cavity or should it include the obliteration of the posterior cavity? This is a question which must be answered by each individual surgeon, the first aim being the patient's safety. Whatever the answer, the cavities managed in this way seem to be much more stable than mastoidectomy cavities, and the results, from a functional point of view, are appreciably better.

Closed Techniques

Difficulty of Performing a Closed-Technique Operation

The difficulty cannot be denied, but it is still comparable to the difficulty which may be encountered when using an open technique correctly. Both require long training. To illustrate the comparability of these difficulties, we shall take as an example the frequency of postoperative facial palsy in our series:

	Immediate FP	Secondary FP
Open technique	0.39%	0.52%
Closed technique	0.18%	0.81%

It must be noted that open techniques are used in cases where the lesions are generally more severe. The estimate of 1% of cases of postoperative total deafness with a closed technique must thus be balanced by an estimate of 2.8% with an open technique. Although some authors, like Jansen, use a closed technique whatever the anatomical situation, we should not hesitate to abandon it in a case of very low dura of the middle fossa or sigmoid sinus in an extremely forward position.

Residual Cholesteatoma

The frequency with which residual cholesteatomas occur may seem disquieting. The surgeon's technical experience will obviously help to reduce this frequency, but there is a certain percentage below which it is difficult to go. This percentage would seem to be 30% for most authors at the present time. This explains our routine planning of a second look. For those authors who do not perform a second-look operation, residual cholesteatoma represents a failure. When it is routinely planned, the existence of a residual cholesteatoma has been foreseen and can therefore be dealt with. The importance of certain techniques must be remembered in connection with the prevention of these residual cholesteatomas. Proper opening of the mastoid allows a large posterior tympanotomy, and a perfect view of the anterior attic. Sacrifice of the tympano-ossicular system is performed as required: removal of the head of the malleus, cutting the tensor tympani tendon, and more if necessary. The cholesteatoma is dissected from behind forwards, from above downwards, and from the edges to the centre in the tympanic cavity, attempting to keep it intact so as to be able to

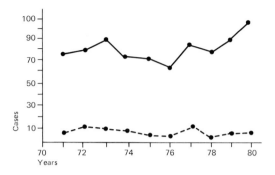

Fig. 82. Frequency of retraction pockets in closed-technique surgery [Deguine's series – thesis by Chuard]: ●——● = 822 closed techniques; ●–––● = 78 retraction pockets.

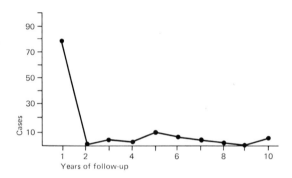

Fig. 83. Time relations of retraction pockets in closed-technique surgery [Deguine's series – thesis by Chuard]: 5% of long-term retraction pockets in a series of 1,071 closed techniques in 10 years.

remove it in one piece. Irrigation must be careful only from behind forwards.

The location of these residual cholesteatomas is interesting to note. They are found essentially in the anterior attic (46%) and in the tympanic cavity (30%), especially in the region of the windows and the facial recess.

Their macroscopic appearance – encapsulated and of medium size in 80% of the cases in our series – is in our view an essential criterion providing an a posteriori justification for the choice of the closed technique, since their complete removal is a certainty. It is more difficult to lay down the approach to be adopted when there is an ill-defined mass of epithelium. In such cases it must be decided whether to perform a third-stage operation, or to transform it into an open technique. The decision will depend on the functional and anatomical situation (oedema of the mucosa, effusion).

Recurrence – the Problem of Retraction Pockets

Retraction pockets appear in approximately 10% of the cases in our combined series (from 8 to 16% in the individual series). In some cases they seem to be an inevitable development. The methods of prevention which we have described in the chapter on surgical techniques may reduce their frequency but cannot eliminate them entirely. We wish to stress the absolute necessity of replacing any substance lost from the bony sulcus. By the application of this principle, the percentage of retraction pockets in the series of one of the present authors dropped from 15 to 6% over 10 years. This series does nonetheless show, although the majority of retraction pockets appear during that the first year, they may also occur at any time during the following 10 years (see chart) (fig. 82, 83). This clearly shows the necessity for regular, lifelong follow-up and inspection. Some of these pockets, being controllable and without collection of debris, remain stable. The others develop and require further surgery which, in some cases, will lead to conversion to an open technique.

Resorption of the Posterior Wall Canal

This has been described by some authors [255, 256]. In our own experience, we have only seen it in exceptional cases, as we avoid excessive thinning of the canal.

Results from a Functional Point of View

The quality of the results, from a functional point of view, of the open or closed techniques, is still a question of some controversy. In an attempt to provide an answer, we have looked at our combined results

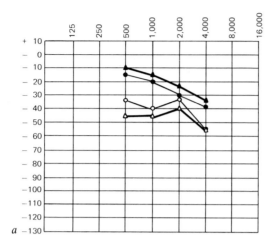

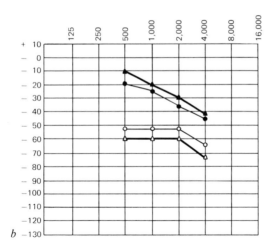

Fig. 84. Average residual air-bone gap preoperatively (▲, △) and postoperatively (●, ○). *a* Open technique with reconstruction of ossicular chain (72 cases). Average residual air-bone gap 17 dB. *b* Open technique without reconstruction of ossicular chain

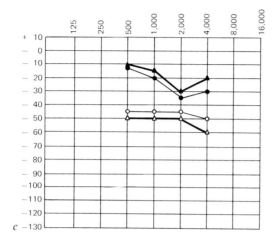

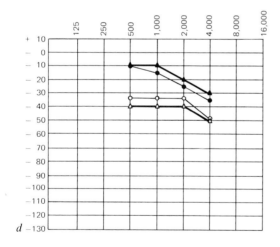

(56 cases). Average residual air-bone gap 25 dB. *c* Closed technique without arch of
stapes (7 cases). Average residual air-bone gap 21 dB. *d* Closed technique with intact
stapes (37 cases). Average residual air-bone gap 12 dB.

in three different ways. The first was set out in detail in the chapter on the results, comparing the gap between the postoperative air conduction and the preoperative bone conduction. The table below gives a slight advantage for the closed technique:

		Open technique	Open technique with obliteration	Closed technique
Intact stapes	AC–BC ≤ 10 dB	17%	30%	37%
	AC–BC ≤ 20 dB	61%	64%	69%
Missing crura	AC–BC ≤ 10 dB	20%	20%	26%
	AC–BC ≤ 20 dB	60%	48%	60%

The second was to consider the development of each case compared to its preoperative state, to appreciate the individual improvement, set out in the table below:

	Number of cases	Improved		Unchanged		Aggravated	
		n	%	n	%	n	%
Open technique	144	70	48.6	46	31.9	28	19.4
Closed technique	503	291	57	179	35.5	33	6.5

This way of looking at the results also justifies the closed techniques.

The third criterion of assessment is the averaging of the audiometric data over a series of 264 cases. The average residual air-bone gap was (fig. 84): (a) 17 dB with an open technique with reconstruction of ossicular chain; (b) 25 dB with an open technique without ossicular reconstruction; (c) 21 dB with a closed technique and ossicular reconstruction on the footplate; (d) 12 dB with a closed technique and reconstruction on intact stapes.

These three methods of comparing open and closed techniques all show the closed technique as advantageous. We recognize that this advantage, although definite, is only slight. It is part of the justification of our preference for the closed technique whenever this is reasonably possible. Nonetheless, whether an open or a closed technique is used, the most satisfactory results, from a functional point of view, are obtained when the ossicular chain is reconstructed in a tympanic cavity with healthy mucosa and a stabilized tympanic membrane and such conditions are often only found, in cholesteatoma cases, when there is a second-look operation.

Report on the Survey

Let us remind the reader that we have only taken into account series containing at least 100 cases, in our view a statistically significant figure. The question of the choice of technique has already been dealt, within the chapter on indications, in which we also reported on authors' attitudes to the second look and the management of the posterior cavity.

Open Techniques

Problems Posed by the Cavity
In the case of the standard radical mastoidectomy, in reply to the question of whether the cavities posed any problem, the authors gave the following answers (in alphabetical order); 50% for Ansart, 43% for Bluestone, 20% for Cotin and Depaepe, 2% for Fisch, 16% for Fleury, 15% for Fombeur, 0% for Gersdorff, 50% for Jansen, 30% for Klein, 20% for Limbour, 24% for Marco, 5% for Martin, 25% for Pech, 10% for Pfaltz, 30% for Sade and Berco, 16% for Sakai, 10% for Sheehy, and 100% for Smyth.

Closure of the tympanic cavity, whether or not it is associated with the management of the posterior cavity, does not appear to affect the instability of the later cavity in the view of the majority of the authors, supprising though this may seem at first sight. For Smyth [635], however, the proportion of unstable cavities drops from 100 to 10% and for Sade and Berco [189] from 30 to 17%; Palva encounters problems in 12% of his cases.

Residual Cholesteatomas
When the tympanic cavity is closed, the proportion of residual cholesteatomas behind the reconstruction is 7% for Bluestone, 26% for Fombeur, 0% for Jansen, 30% for Klein, 20% for Limbour, 24% for

Marco, 25% for Pech, 1% for Sakai, and 2% for Sheehy. Smyth finds 13% in the tympanic cavity and 17% in the attic. Palva reports 6.4% in the tympanic cavity after 10 years.

We have very little information for cases where the posterior cavity is obliterated or lined with a flap, since the authors rarely have a second look in these cases. In a series of 100 cases with a routine second look between 5 and 12 months after the operation, Smyth [635] only observed one pearl in the posterior cavity. For Tos, 2% of residual cholesteatomas appear subsequently, beneath the obliteration.

Closed Techniques

Residual Cholesteatomas

Greatly varying percentages are reported, from 5% for Sakai to 80% for Depaepe. It must be stressed that these figures for residual cholesteatomas must be interpreted in the light of the extent to which the second look is routine. Although Smyth, for example, now performs a routine second-look operation in 100% of his cases, Jansen will only do so if forced into it. The second look is planned in 100% of cases for Zini, 75% for Fisch, 56% for Bluestone, 45% for Gersdorff, 42% for Fombeur, and 14% for Pech.

When a residual cholesteatoma is found, the authors' attitudes generally depend on the macroscopic appearance. If there is a well-defined, moderately sized pearl, most surgeons remove it, preserving the posterior canal wall and, in some cases, planning a third look (Smyth, Fisch). When the epithelial formation is diffuse, most of the surgeons questioned change to an open technique (Ansart, Fisch, Martin, Pech, Pfaltz, Vergnon).

Retraction Pocket

This appears in 12% of cases for Fisch, 38% for Tos, 25% for Jansen, 29% for Fombeur, and 17% for Zini. Development into a cholesteatoma is variable: 2% for Tos, 15% for Jansen, 17% for Fombeur, 12% for Fisch, and 8% for Zini (these figures are given as percentages of the total number of operations, and not as a percentage of the total number of retraction pockets). When a retraction pocket is found, the surgeons' attitudes are generally less conservative than when a residual pearl is found. Although Jansen maintains a closed technique, such authors as Austin, Fombeur and Smyth change to an open technique. Zini maintains a closed technique in 64% of his cases, changes to an open technique in 34%, and performs a standard radical mastoidectomy in 12% of these.

Results from a Functional Point of View

The colleagues whom we questioned did not answer this question in precise detail, but rather gave us their general impressions. Most of them find no appreciable difference between open and closed techniques (Pech, Tos, Sakai, Smyth). Bremond, Fisch, Sheehy, Gersdorff, Ansart and Zini all expressed a preference for the closed technique. As we have already stated, Jansen uses almost exclusively the closed technique, and functional improvement is not the most important point for him.

The advantage of using a closed technique with children is shown by Naclerio et al. [148], who report that hearing improves in 50% of operations on children, and 30% for adults. For Smyth, the air-bone gap is less than 11 dB in the following percentages of cases: (a) 90% when the ossicular chain is intact; (b) 75% when a bone graft is placed between the malleus and the superstructure of the stapes; (c) 65% when the graft is placed between the tympanic membrane and the superstructure of the stapes, and (d) 55% when a cartilage is placed between the tympanic membrane and the footplate. For Fleury, using an open technique, the air-bone gap is less than 20 dB in 20% of the cases in a series of 165 operations.

General Impressions

We were struck by the desire of many authors to carry out preventive treatment on the cholesteatoma while still at the retraction pocket stage (Sakai, Smyth, Sterkers). As for the treatment of the fully-developed cholesteatoma, there seem to be three main attitudes to future trends: (1) Some surgeons, disappointed by the closed technique, are turning, or returning, to the open techniques (Fombeur, Gersdorff, Smyth, Depaepe). They take their places beside those who, like Fleury, Palmgren and Ansart, have always preferred open techniques in the majority of cases. Amongst these surgeons, the attitude towards obliteration is also changing. Some, such as Palva, Palmgren and Montandon, continue to obliterate. Others, such as Sakai, are tending to abandon it, or use the technique sparingly, like Smyth. (2) Others, on the other hand, such as Bremond and Zini, are joining Jansen, Marquet and Sterkers in showing a marked preference for the closed technique. (3) A large number of surgeons continue to adopt an electic approach, with which we are in entire agreement. These include Fisch, Portmann, Sheehy, and Tos.

Opinions differ as regards children. Sheehy and Smyth adopt exactly the same approach as with adults. Some authors favour, and consistently use, closed techniques with children (Crabtee, Austin, Schuknecht, Derlacki, Bluestone, Gersdorff, Perkins). The degree of pneumatization is the main factor which, depending on the diathesis, should put the surgeon on his guard against an unstable cavity. All the authors combine this technique with a routine second look. Some surgeons, however, such as Andrieu-Guitrancourt, Pech, Farrior and Poncet, choose in certain cases to use an open technique on children.

Conclusions

The appearance of a cholesteatoma in the middle ear is, in most cases, only one aspect of the development of a dysfunction of the Eustachian tube, which is the cause of the majority of chronic inflammatory infections of the middle ear, although other main or subsidiary mechanisms may also come into play. The surgical treatment of the cholesteatoma is thus only one stage in the treatment of a disease which begins in childhood and whose most characteristic manifestation is seromucous otitis.

The prophylactic treatment of the cholesteatoma thus begins at this stage with curing the seromucous otitis: by adenoidectomy, anti-inflammatory treatment, crenotherapy or transtympanic aeration. Above all, regular microscope examination over a long period is necessary to check for the possible appearance of a retraction pocket, which is a veritable precursor of cholesteatoma. If one is discovered, medical treatment, the most effective elements of which are crenotherapy and the insertion of a transtympanic aeration tube, should be intensified. If such treatment fails, surgery, as we have described it, must be resorted to.

The surgical treatment of the fully developed cholesteatoma was rejuvenated 20 years ago with the introduction of the closed techniques. These introduced a new degree of thoroughness in the eradication of the lesions, and the aim of reconstructing a middle ear which is as close as possible to normal, both from an anatomical and from a functional point of view. With experience, we can now appreciate both the achievements and the failures of this type of operation. Two causes of failure in particular have been the subject of much discussion – residual cholesteatoma and recurrence through a retraction pocket.

Residual cholesteatoma can be dealt with by the thorough surgical technique we have described, and by the routine second look which we advocate. True recurrence through a retraction pocket on the other hand, seems to be impossible to control in some cases; it provides evidence that the tubal dysfunction persists, and seems to be the final barrier for the closed techniques. Moreover, the use of the closed technique has had the immense advantage of bringing new life to the performance of open-technique tympanoplasty, by applying the same principles of thorough eradication and reconstruction of the tympano-ossicular system. Seen in this light, the open technique, which might seem easier to perform, in fact requires the same experience and thoroughness as the closed technique.

In any event, the surgical treatment is only one stage. Whichever technique is adopted, long-term follow-up and inspection at regular intervals is essential.

We have attempted to be objective in drawing up this report, since as we all know, 'whatever is exaggerated cannot be believed' (Paul Valéry).

References

1 Aboulker, P.; Demaldent, J.B.; Pelisse, J.M.: Réflexions sur le cholestéatome. Annls. Oto-lar. *92:*277–292 (1975).

2 Aboulker, P.; Demaldent, J.E.; Manach, Y.: Problèmes thérapeutiques de l'otite chronique et de ses séquelles sur oreille fonctionnellement unique. Annls. Oto-lar. *95:*269–279 (1978).

3 Abramson, M.: Collagenolytic activity in middle ear cholesteatoma. Ann. Otol. *78:* 112–125 (1969).

4 Abramson, M.; Chen-Chung, H.: Localization of collagenase in human middle ear cholesteatoma. Laryngoscope *87:*771–791 (1977).

5 Abramson, M.; Chen-Chung, H.: Cholesteatoma and bone resorption. 1st Int. Conf. on Middle Ear Cholesteatome, Iowa 1977 (Aesculapius, Birmingham 1977).

6 Abramson, M.; Gross, J.: Further studies on a collagenase in middle ear cholesteatoma. Ann. Otol. *80:*177–185 (1971).

7 Abramson, M.; Harker, L.A., McCabe, B.F.: Labyrinthine fistula complicating chronic suppurative otitis media. Archs Otolar. *100:*141–142 (1974).

8 Alberti, P.W.R.M.: Epithelial migration on the tympanic membrane. J. Lar. Otol. *78:*808 (1964).

9 Andrea, M.: Regiaio posterior da caixa do timpano. Estudo anatomo-cirurgico; thèse Lisbonne (1975).

10 Andrieu-Guitrancourt, J.; Dehesdin, D.; Schlosser, M.: Traitement de l'otite moyenne chronique cholestéatomateuse de l'enfant. Annls. Oto-lar. *97:*39–44 (1980).

11 Anson, J.B.; Donaldson, A.J.: The surgical anatomy of the temporal bone and ear (Saunders, Philadelphia, 1973).

12 Antoli-Candella, F.: Audiocururgia de la otorreas y de sus secuelas. Ponencia Official VII Congresso National ORL (1972).

13 Austin, D.F.: The retraction pocket in the treatment of cholesteatoma. Archs Otolar. *102:*741–743 (1976).

14 Austin, D.F.: The significance of retraction pocket in the treatment of cholesteatoma. 1st Int. Conf. on Middle Ear Cholesteatoma, Iowa 1977 (Aesculapius, Birmingham 1977).

15 Baron, S.H.: Preservation of the cholesteatoma matrix in the modified radical mastoidectomy. Laryngoscope *61:*(1967).

16 Barrault, S.: Voie d'abord chirurgical d'abord du sinus tympani; thèse Paris (1980).

17 Beaumont, G.D.: Cholesterol granuloma. J. otolar. Soc. Aust. *2:*28–35 (1967).

18 Bernstein, J.M.; Hausmann, E.; Wright, J.: Middle ear disease release of soluble factors stimulating bone resorption. 1st Int. Conf. on Middle Ear Cholesteatome, Iowa 1977 (Aesculapius, Birmingham, 1977).

19 Bluestone, C.D.; Beery, Q.C.: Concepts in the pathogenesis of middle ear effu-sions. Ann. Otol. *85:*suppl. 25, p. 182 (1976).

20 Bluestone, C.D., Cantekin, E.I.; Beery, Q.S.; Douglas, G.S.; Stool, S.E.: Func-tional Eustachian tube obstruction in acquired cholesteatoma and related condi-tions. 1st Int. Conf. on Middle Ear Cholesteatome, Iowa 1977 (Aesculapius, Bir-mingham 1977).

21 Bluestone, C.D.; Casselbrant, M.L.; Cantekin, E.I.: Functional obstruction of the Eustachian tube in the pathogenesis of aural cholesteatoma in children; in Choles-teatoma and mastoid surgery (Kugler, Amsterdam, 1982).

22 Bodelet, B.; Wayoff, M.: Notes préliminaires sur l'ultrastructure du cholestéatome. Annls. Oto-lar. *87:* 449 (1970).

23 Bouche, J.; Freche, C.; François, J.: Otites moyennes chroniques. EMC ORL, Paris 1, 20095 (1964).

24 Bremond, G.; Magnan, J.: Eradication du cholestéatome et chirurgie réparatrice de l'oreille moyenne. Cah. ORL *14:* 289–294 (1979).

25 Bremond, G.; Magnan, J.: Evolution et critique des idées concernant le cholesté-atome. J. fr. ORL *30:* 25–30 (1981).

26 Bremond, G.; Magnan, J.; Acquaviva, F.: Cholestéatome et métaplasie épidermoïde. Différences et similitudes. Acta oto-rhino-lar. belg. *34:* 34–42 (1980).

27 Bremond, G.; Magnan, J.; De Micco, M.: Les aspects microscopiques du choles-téatome. Cah. ORL *10:* 303–311 (1975).

28 Bremond, G.; Wayoff, M.; Jost, G.: Les étapes du traitement de l'otite chronique chez l'adulte. Rapport Sté Fse d'ORL et pathologie cervico-faciale (Arnette, Paris 1966).

29 Buckingham, R.A.: Cholesteatoma and chronic otitis media following middle ear intubation. Laryngoscope *91:* 1450–1471 (1981).

30 Bumsted, R.; Dolan, K.; Sade, J.; McCabe, B.: Preservation of cochlear function after extensive labyrinthine destruction. Ann. Otol. *86:* 131 (1977).

31 Cantekin, E.I.; Bluestone, C.D.; Parkin, L.: Eustachian tube ventilatory function in children. Ann. Otol. *85:*suppl. 25, 171 (1976).

32 Cawthorne, T.: Congenital cholesteatoma. Archs Otolar. *78:* 248 (1963).

33 Charachon, R.: Evidements, tympanoplasties EMC ORL Paris, 20.110 A10, A20, A30 (1977).

34 Charachon, R.: Cholesteatoma, epidermization: choice between closed and obli-teration technique. Clin. Otolaryngol. *3:* 363–367 (1978).

35 Charachon, R.: Cholestéatome intra-pétreux. Revue Lar. Otol. Rhinol. *100:* 119–123 (1979).

36 Charachon, R.; Couderc, P.; Junien-Lavillauroy, C.: Les tympanoplasties – anato-mie pathologique. Cah. ORL *12:* 397–442 (1977).

37 Charachon, R.; Eyraud, S.; Guenoun, A.; Egal, F.: The surgical treatment of cho-lesteatoma in children. Clin. Otolaryngol. *10:* 177–184 (1985).

38 Charachon, R.; Junien-Lavillauroy, C.; Accoyer, B.; Serero, C.; Suard, J.C.: Tolér-ance clinique du silastic par l'oreille moyenne: son intérêt dans les tympanoplasties en deux temps. R.M.A.F *3:* 438–444 (1974).

39 Charachon, R.; Roux, O.: La suppression du cholestéatome du sinus tympani et de la gouttière postérieure de la caisse. J. fr. ORL *30:* 191–194 (1981).

40 Charachon, R.; Roux, O.; Dumas, G.: Les cholestéatomes à tympan fermé de l'oreille moyenne et du rocher. J.fr. ORL *30:* 157 (1981).
41 Charachon, R.; Roux, O.; Dumas, G.: Les cholestéatomes iatrogènes de l'oreille moyenne: étiologie et prévention. J.fr. ORL *30:* 235 (1981).
42 Charachon, R.; Roux, O.; Eyraud, S.: Le cholestéatome de l'oreille moyenne. Choix des techniques et résultats chez l'adulte et chez l'enfant. Annls. Oto-lar. *97:* 65–78 (1980).
43 Chole, R.A.; MacGinn, M.D.; Henry, K.R.: The gerbilline cholesteatoma; in Cholesteatoma and mastoid surgery (Kugler, Amsterdam, 1982).
44 Chouard, C.H.; Charachon, R.; Morgon, A.; Cathala, H.P.: Anatomie, pathologie et chirurgie du nerf facial (Masson, Paris 1972).
45 Chuard, P.: Le cholestéatome de l'oreille moyenne (à propos d'une étude informatisée sur 1071 cas); thèse Lille (1982).
46 Claes, J.; Marquet, J.F.E.: Cholesteatomatous invasion of the middle ear: classical points of entrance and their pathways; in Surgery and pathology of the middle ear (Nijhoff, Antwerp 1985).
47 Cody, D.: The definition of cholesteatoma. 1st Int. Conf. on Middle Ear Cholesteatoma, Iowa 1977 (Aesculapius, Birmingham 1977).
48 Curtis, A.W.: Congenital middle ear cholesteatoma: two unusual cases and a review of the literature. Laryngoscope *89:* 1159–1165 (1979).
49 Deguine, C.: Long-term results in cholesteatoma surgery. Clin. Otolaryngol. *3:* 301–310 (1978).
50 Deguine, C.: Prévention de la récidive du cholestéatome dans les techniques fermées. 75e Congr. Sté Fse ORL et pathologie cervico-faciale (Arnette, Paris 1978).
51 Deguine, C.: Le traitement chirurgical du cholestéatome en technique fermée. Annls. Oto-lar. *97:* 99–103 (1980).
52 Deguine, C.; Desaulty, A.: Le traitement du cholestéatome de l'oreille moyenne. Indication de la chirurgie ouverte et fermée. 71è Congr. Sté Fse ORL et pathologie cervico-faciale (Arnette, Paris 1974).
53 Deguine, C.; Desaulty, A.: La réparation du conduit osseux dans la chirurgie du cholestéatome. Revue Larg. Otol. Rhinol. *105:* 461–463 (1984).
54 Derlacki, E.L.: Etiological aspects in congenital cholesteatoma. 1st Int. Conf. on Middle Ear Cholesteatome, Iowa 1977 (Aesculapius, Birmingham 1977).
55 Derlacki, E.L.: Congenital cholesteatoma of the middle ear and mastoid: a fourth report. Proc. 5th Shambaugh Int. Workshop on Middle Ear Surgery, 1976.
56 Derlacki, E.L.; Clemis, J.D.: Congenital cholesteatoma of the middle ear and mastoid. Ann. Otol. *74:* 706 (1965).
57 Diamant, M.; Diamant, H.: The mastoid hair cells. 1st Int. Conf. on Middle Ear Cholesteatoma, Iowa 1977 (Aesculapius, Birmingham 1977).
58 Donaldson, J.; Anson, J.B.; Warpeka, R.L.; Rensink, M.J.: The surgical anatomy of the sinus tympani. Archs Otolar. *91:* 219–227 (1970).
59 Eden, A.R.: Glomus tympanicum: implications for a middle ear aeration reflex; in Cholesteatoma and mastoid surgery (Kugler, Amsterdam 1982).
60 Egal, F.: Le traitement chirurgical du cholestéatome de l'enfant; thèse Grenoble (1984).
61 Elbaze, D.: La tympanoplastie en technique ouverte avec comblement musculo-périosté: modalités, techniques, résultats, indications; thèse Grenoble (1983).

62 Eliachar, I.; Joachims, H.Z.: Arrest of cholesteatoma formation by long-term ven-
    tilation of the middle ear; in Cholesteatoma and mastoid surgery (Kugler, Amster-
    dam 1982).
63 Elnar, A.; Ingelstedt, S.; Ivarsson, A.: Indirect determination of the middle ear
    pressure. Acta oto-lar. 72: 255 (1971).
64 Escher, F.: Traumatic cholesteatoma of the middle ear. Acta oto-lar. 50: 47–52
    (1959).
65 Falk, B.: Tubal dysfunction in patients with cleft palate; in Cholesteatoma and
    mastoid surgery (Kugler, Amsterdam 1982).
66 Eviatar, A.; Jamal, H.: Cholesteatoma induced by stapedectomy. Archs Otolar.
    109: 413–414 (1983).
67 Feldmann, H.: Eine Stichsäge für die Mikrochirurgie – neue Möglichkeiten zu
    osteoplastischen Eingriffen am Ohr und den Nebenhöhlen. Arch. Ohr.-Nas.-
    KehlkHeilk. 216: 2 (1977).
68 Feldmann, H.: Surgeon's workshop: osteoplastic approach in chronic otitis media by
    means of a microsurgical reciprocating saw. Clin. Otolaryngol. 3: 515–520 (1978).
69 Fernandez, C.; Lindsay, J.; Moskowitz, M.: Some observations on the pathogene-
    sis of middle ear cholesteatoma. Archs. Otolar. 69: 537–546 (1959).
70 Fernandez, C.; Lindsay, J.R.: Aural cholesteatoma. Experimental observations.
    Laryngoscope 70: 1119 (1960).
71 Fisch, U.: 'Congenital' cholesteatoma of the supra-labyrinthine region. Clin. Oto-
    laryngol. 3: 369–376 (1978).
72 Fisch, U.: Tympanoplasty and stapedectomy. A manual of techniques (Thieme,
    Stuttgart 1980).
73 Fisch, U.: Intracranial complications of cholesteatoma; in Cholesteatoma and
    mastoid surgery (Kugler, Amsterdam 1982).
74 Fleischer, K.: Die Entwicklungsgeschichte der schrapnellschen Membran. Arch.
    Ohr.-Nas.-KehlkHeilk. 164: 434–453 (1953).
75 Fleury, P.; Basset, J.M.; Brasnu, D.; Compère, J.F.; Pansier, P.: L'évidement: ta-
    bou de l'otite chronique cholestéatomateuse. Notre opinion basée sur une expéri-
    ence personnelle. Annls Oto-lar. 97: 35–38 (1980).
76 Fleury, P.; Basset, J.M.; Coupez, D.; Compère, J.F.: L'otite chronique ostéoma-
    teuse. Annls Oto-lar. 95: 665–675 (1978).
77 Fleury, P.; Legent, F.; Lefebvre, C.: Atlas des techniques chirurgicales de l'oreille
    (Masson, Paris 1974).
78 Fleury, P.; Thibaut, B.; Lefeure, C.: Le traitement des lésions du récessus facial
    suprapyramidal au cours de certaines otites chroniques. Annls Oto-lar. 90: 475–480
    (1973).
79 Forni, J.F.: Analyse informatique des interventions pour 400 cholestéatomes de
    l'oreille moyenne; thèse Nancy (1979).
80 Fombeur, J.P.; Bouton, V.; Dobler, S.: Evaluation des différentes techniques utili-
    sées dans le traitement des cholestéatomes. Annls Oto-lar. 97: 85–89 (1980).
81 Freeman, P.: Fistula of the lateral semi-circular canal. Clin. Otolaryngol. 3:
    315–322 (1978).
82 Friedman, I.: The pathology of epidermoid cholesteatoma – human and experi-
    mental. 1st Int. Conf. on Middle Ear Cholesteatoma, Iowa 1977 (Aesculapius, Bir-
    mingham 1977).

83 Gacek, R.R.: The surgical management of labyrinthine fistulae in chronic otitis media with cholesteatoma. Ann. Otol. suppl. 10 (1974).

84 Gacek, R.R.: Diagnosis and management of primary tumors of the petrous apex. Ann. Otol., suppl. 18 (1975).

85 Gacek, R.R.: Mastoid and middle ear cavity obliteration for control of otitis media. Ann. Otol. 85: 305–309 (1976).

86 Gaillard, J.; Haguenauer, J.P.; Dumolard, P.; Romanet, P.; Dubreuil, C.: Cholestéatome post-traumatique du conduit et de l'oreille moyenne. J. fr. ORL 25: 491–492 (1976).

87 Gans, H.; Wlodyka, J.: Mastoid pneumatization in chronic otitis media. Archs Otolar. 83: 343–346 (1966).

88 Gantz, B.J.; Maynard, J.: Ultrastructural evaluation of biochemical events of bone resorption in human chronic otitis media. Am. J. Otol. 3: 279–283 (1982).

89 Georges, B.; Roux, F.; Cophignon, J.: Abcès du cerveau. La ponction est-elle suffisante? Concours méd. 103: 6046–6050 (1981).

90 Gersdorff, M.C.H.; Hamoir, M.: Notre expérience dans la chirurgie du cholestéatome. Acta oto-rhino-lar. belg. 36: 382–392 (1982).

91 Gersdorff, M.C.H.; Maisin, J.P.: Management of the retro-tympanum; in Surgery and pathology of the middle ear (Nijhoff, Antwerp 1985).

92 Girard, L.: Atlas d'anatomie et de médecine opératoire du labyrinthe osseux (Maloine, Paris 1939).

93 Glasgold, A.I.: Cholesteatoma following myringotomy and ventilation tube. Eye Ear Nose Throat Mon. 53: 274–275 (1974).

94 Glasscock, M.E.: Results in cholesteatoma surgery. 1st Int. Conf. on Middle Ear Cholesteatoma, Iowa 1977 (Aesculapius, Birmingham 1977).

95 Glasscock, M.E.; Miller, G.W.: Intact canal wall tympanoplasty in the management of cholesteatoma. Laryngoscope 86: 1639–1657 (1976).

96 Goedbloed, J.F.: The early development of the middle ear. Archs Biol., Liège 75: 207–243 (1964).

97 Goodhill, V.: A cholesteatoma chronicle. Archs Otolar. 97: 183 (1973).

98 Goodhill, V.: Ear diseases (Harper & Row, New York 1979).

99 Gristwood, R.E.: Chronic otitis media with epidermoid cholesteatoma. A discussion of some points of controversy concerning surgical management. Clin. Otolaryngol. 1: 337–342 (1976).

100 Guerrier, Y.; Andrea, M.; Biancalana, G.: Région postérieure de la caisse du tympan et systématisation. Cah. ORL 11: 779–792 (1976).

101 Guerrier, Y.; Andrea, M.; Paco, J.: Les repaires anatomiques du cholestéatome dans la caisse du tympan. Annls Oto-lar. 97: 15–28 (1980).

102 Harell, M.: Prevalence of cholesteatoma in black Americans; in Cholesteatoma and mastoid surgery (Kugler, Amsterdam 1982).

103 Harris, H.J.: Cholesteatosis and chronic otitis media. Laryngoscope 72: 954 (1962).

104 Haussmann, E.: Structural requirements of bone resorption by endoxin and lipoteichoic acid. J. dent. Res. 54: 94–99 (1975).

105 Holmquist, J.; Lindeman, P.: Tympanometric studies in cholesteatoma and retraction pockets; in Cholesteatoma and mastoid surgery (Kugler, Amsterdam 1982).

106 Honda, Y.: Acquired and recurrent cholesteatoma; in Surgery and pathology of the middle ear (Nijhoff, Antwerp 1985).

107 Horton, J.F.: Bone resorption activity in supernatant fluid from cultural human peripheral blood lymphocytes. Science *177:*793–795 (1972).

108 House, J.W.; Sheehy, J.L.: Cholesteatoma with intact tympanic membrane: a report of 41 cases. Laryngoscope *90:*70–75 (1980).

109 Jackson, D.G.; Lim, D.J.: Fine morphology of the advancing front of cholesteatoma – experimental and human. Acta oto-lar. *86:*71–88 (1978).

110 Jahnke, V.; Falk, W.: Clinical, pathological and therapeutic aspects of cholesteatoma in children. Lar. Rhinol. Otol. *55:*556–560 (1976).

111 Jansen, C.: Canal wall up tympanoplasty for cholesteatoma. Proc. 6th Shambaugh Int. Workshop on Otomicrosurgery, Chicago 1960.

112 Jansen, C.: Posterior tympanotomy access to the middle ear with preservation of the external canal. Arch. Ohr.-Nas.-KehlkHeilk. *188:*558–559 (1967).

113 Jansen, C.: Über Radikaloperation und Tympanoplastik. Sber. Fortbild. Ärztek. (1958).

114 Jansen, C.: The combined approach for tympanoplasty (report of 10 years' experience). J. Lar. Otol. *82:*779 (1968).

115 Jansen, C.: Evaluation of surgery for cholesteatoma. 1st Int. Conf. on Middle Ear Cholesteatoma, Iowa 1977 (Aesculapius, Birmingham 1977).

116 Jansen, C.: Cholesteatoma in children. Clin. Otolaryngol. *3:*349–352 (1978).

117 Jansen, C.: Combined approach tympanoplasty in cholesteatoma surgery: a report on 1,904 adults and on 472 children; in Cholesteatoma and mastoid surgery (Kugler, Amsterdam 1982).

118 Jansen, C.: Preservation of the auditory canal: a surgical procedure for everybody; in Cholesteatoma and mastoid surgery (Kugler, Amsterdam 1982).

119 Kaneko, Y. et al.: Bone destruction due to the rupture of a cholesteatoma sac: a pathogenesis of bone destruction in aural cholesteatoma. Laryngoscope *90:* 1865–1871 (1980).

120 Klein, D.; Rais, Z.L.: Prostaglandins: stimulation of bone resorption in tissue culture. Endocrinology *14:*36–40 (1970).

121 Kluyskens, P.; Gillis, E.; Insabumukunzi, S.: First observation on treatment of cholesteatoma with (N-acetyl)cysteine. Acta oto-lar. *87:*362–365 (1979).

122 Koch, U.; Straehler-Pohl, H.J.: Post-operative epitympanale Trommelfellretraktion beim Cholesteatom. Lar. Rhinol. Otol. *60:*654–657 (1981).

123 Kolihova, E.; Abraham, J.; Blashova, O.: Rezidivierende Mittelohrentzündung im frühen Kindesalter und ihr Einfluss auf die Zellsystementwicklung des Schläfenbeins. Radiologe *12:*62–68 (1972).

124 Lacher, G.: Les récidives de cholestéatome post-opératoires en chirurgie tympanoplastique. Revue Lar. Otol. Rhinol., extr. 7–8 (1970).

125 Lim, D.J.; Birck, H.G.; Saunders, W.H.: Aural cholesteatoma and epidermization: a fine morphological study. 1st Int. Conf. on Middle Ear Cholesteatoma Surgery, Iowa 1977 (Aesculapius, Birmingham 1977).

126 Lim, D.J.; Saunders, W.H.: Acquired cholesteatoma: light and electronic microscopic observation. Ann. Otol. *81:*2–12 (1972).

127 Link, R.: Die Bedeutung des Cutisstreiftens bei der Entwicklung eines Mittelohrcholesteatoms. Acta oto-lar. *49:*411–420 (1958).

128 Linthicum, F.H.: Cholesterol granuloma (iatrogenic): further evidence of etiology – A case report. Ann. Otol. *80:*207 (1971).

129 Litton, W.B.: Epithelial migration over tympanic membrane and external canal. Archs Otolar. *77:* 254–257 (1963).

130 Litton, W.B.: Epidermal migration in the ear: the location and characteristics of the generation center revealed by utilizing a radioactive desoxyribose nucleic-acid precursor. Acta oto-lar., suppl. 240 (1968).

131 Maduro, R.: Les suppurations chroniques de l'orcille (l'Expansion scientifique française, Paris 1965).

132 Magnan, J.: Le cholestéatome – Notions actuelles; thèse Marseille (1972).

133 Magnuson, B.: Tubal closing failure in retraction type cholesteatoma and adhesive middle ear lesions. Acta oto-lar. *86:* 408–417 (1978).

134 Magnuson, B.: The atelectatic ear. Int. J. pediat. Otolar. *3:* 25–35 (1981).

135 Magnuson, B.: Tympanoplasty and recurrent disease. Am. J. Otol. *2:* 277–283 (1981).

136 Magnuson, B.: Tubal opening and closing ability in unilateral middle ear disease. Am. J. Otol. *2:* 199–209 (1981).

137 Magnuson, B.: Retraction type middle ear disease; in Cholesteatoma and mastoid surgery (Kugler, Amsterdam 1982).

138 Marquet, J.: Quelques problèmes particuliers se rapportant aux homogreffes tympano-ossiculaires. Acta oto-rhino-lar. belg. *24:* 4 (1970).

139 Marquet, J.: Cholesteatoma or keratoma. A pathological approach. Acta oto-rhino-lar. belg. *34:* 5–11 (1980).

140 Marquet, J.; Van de Heynink, P.: Cholesteatoma or keratoma: a pathological approach. Belg. Tijdschr. Radiol. *63:* 251–258 (1980).

141 Martin, C.; Martin, H.: Cholestéatome, amputation du promontoire et persistance de reliquats auditifs. J. fr. ORL *27:* 133–134 (1978).

142 Martin, C.; Martin, H.; Michalet, J.F.: Les cholestéatomes du rocher à expansion majeure. A propos de 17 cas. Annls. Oto-lar. *101:* 77–93 (1984).

143 Martin, H.; Morgon, A.; Martin, C.: Caisses réduites et petites caisses (commentaires sur un film). Revue Lar. Otol. Rhinol. *99:* 65–72 (1978).

144 McCabe, B.F.: The incidence, site, treatment and fate of labyrinthine fistula. Clin. Otolaryngol. *3:* 239–242 (1978).

145 McGuckin, F.: Non-malignant destructive ear disease. Archs Otolar. *78:* 358–363 (1963).

146 Mawson, S.R.: Diseases of the ear (Williams & Wilkins, Baltimore 1979).

147 Montandon, P.; Smolik, J.C.: Oblitération radicale des cavités d'évidement pétro-mastoïdien avec tissu adipeux. Problèmes actuels d'ORL (Huber, Bern 1981).

148 Naclerio, L.; Neely, J.G.; Alford, B.R.: A retrospective analysis of the intact canal wall tympanoplasty with mastoidectomy. Am. J. Otol. *2:* 315–317 (1981).

149 Nager, F.R.: The cholesteatoma of the middle ear. Ann. Otol. *34:* 1249 (1925).

150 Nager, G.T.: Epidermoids involving the temporal bone: clinical, radiological and pathological aspects. Laryngoscope *85:* suppl. 2 (1975).

151 Neely, J.G.: Complications of suppurative otitis media (American Academy of Ophthalmology and Otalaryngology, Rochester 1978).

152 Ojala, K.; Palva, A.: Late results of obliterative cholesteatoma surgery. Archs Oto-lar. 1–3 (1982).

153 Palmgren, O.: Long-term results of open cavity and tympanomastoid surgery of the chronic ear. Acta oto-lar. *88:* 343–349 (1979).

154 Palva, T.: A new approach to radical surgery of the chronic otitis media. Practica oto-rhino-lar. *24:*372–382 (1962).

155 Palva, T.: Nonmalignant destructive ear disease. Archs Otolar. *78:*358 (1963).

156 Palva, T.: Chronic otitis media – obliterative techniques; in Surgery and pathology of the middle ear (Nijhoff, Antwerp 1985).

157 Palva, T.; Karma, P.; Palva, A.: Cholesteatoma surgery canal wall down and mastoid obliteration. 1st Int. Conf. on Middle Ear Cholesteatoma, Iowa 1977 (Aesculapius, Birmingham 1977).

158 Palva, T.; Karja, J.; Palva, A.: Opening of the labyrinth during chronic ear surgery. Archs Otolar. *93:*75 (1971).

159 Palva, T.; Makinen, J.: Why does middle ear cholesteatoma recur? Archs Otolar. *109:*513–518 (1983).

160 Palva, T.; Palva, A.; Samivalli, A.: Radical mastoidectomy with cavity obliteration. Archs Otolar. *88:*119 (1968).

161 Paparella, M.M.; Kim, C.S.: Mastoidectomy update. Laryngoscope *87:* 1977–1988 (1977).

162 Peron, D.L.; Schuknecht, H.F.: Congenital cholesteatoma with other abnormalities. Archs. Otolar. *101:*498–505 (1975).

163 Pfaltz, C.R.; Pfaltz, R.; Finkenzeller, P.: Short- and long-term results in ossiculoplasty in cholesteatomatous ears; in Cholesteatoma and mastoid surgery (Kugler, Amsterdam 1982).

164 Pfaltz, C.R.; Pfaltz, R.; Schmidt, P.: Reconstructive surgery in chronic otitis media. Statistical analysis of long-term results. ORL *37:*257–270 (1975).

165 Pfaltz, C.R.; Redli, M.: Occult cholesteatoma of the middle ear. ORL *40:* 23–31 (1978).

166 Piepergerdes, J.C.; Kramer, B.M.; Behnke, E.E.: Keratosis obturans and external auditory canal cholesteatoma. Laryngoscope *90:* 383–391 (1980).

167 Plester, D.: Chirurgie des cholesteatomes. Arch. ORL, Berlin *223:* 380–390 (1979).

168 Plester, D.: The anthropological aspects of Eustachian tube malfunction; in Cholesteatoma and mastoid surgery (Kugler, Amsterdam 1982).

169 Portmann, M.: 'Open' or 'closed' technique surgery of the middle ear. Ann. Otol. *77:*927 (1968).

170 Portmann, M.: Traité de technique chirurgicale ORL et cervico-faciale, vol. 1 (Masson, Paris, 1975).

171 Portmann, M.: Definition of success and failure in cholesteatoma surgery; in Cholesteatoma and mastoid surgery (Kugler, Amsterdam 1982).

172 Portmann, M.; Sterkers, J.M.; Charachon, R.; Chouard, C.H.: Cholestéatome du conduit auditif interne; in Le conduit auditif interne (Arnette, Paris 1973).

173 Proctor, B.: The development of the middle ear spaces and their surgical significance. J. Lar. Otol. *78:*631 (1964).

174 Proctor, B.: Surgical anatomy of the posterior tympanum. Ann. Otol. *5:* 1026–1040 (1969).

175 Proctor, B.: L'ensemble attique-aditus et diaphragme tympanique. Ann. Otol. *80:* 371–375 (1971).

176 Ritter, F.N.: Chronic suppurative otitis media and the pathologic labyrinthine fistula. Laryngoscope *80:* 1025 (1970).

177 Riu, R.; Flottes, L.; Bouche, J.; Leden, R.: La physiologie de la trompe d'Eustache (Arnette, Paris, 1966).

178 Roulleau, P.; Peynegre, R.: Les difficultés thérapeutiques que nous rencontrons au cours des tympanoplasties. Annls. Oto-lar. 97: 91–98 (1980).

179 Roulleau, P.; Peynegre, R.; Receveur, M.; Meme-François, M.: L'abord chirurgical du sinus tympani. Technique ct indications. Sté de Laryngologie des Hôpitaux de Paris, 1980.

180 Roulleau, P.; Peynegre, R.; Receveur, M.; Barrault, S.; Strunski, V.: Evolution de nos techniques au cours des tympanoplasties par homogreffes pour otite chronique cholestéatomateuse ou non. Sté de Laryngologie des Hôpitaux de Paris, 1980.

181 Ruedi, L.: Pathogenesis and treatment of cholesteatoma in chronic suppuration of the temporal bone. Ann. Otol. 66: 283–306 (1957).

182 Ruedi, L.: Cholesteatoma formation in the middle ear in animal experiments. Acta oto-lar. 50: 233–242 (1959).

183 Ruedi, L.: Pathogenesis and surgical treatment of the middle ear cholesteatoma. Acta oto-lar., suppl. 361, pp. 5–45 (1978).

184 Sade, J.: Epithelial invasion of intraossicular spaces. J. Lar. Otol. 86: 15 (1972).

185 Sade, J.: Pathogenesis of attic cholesteatoma. J. R. Soc. Med. 71: 716–732 (1978).

186 Sade, J.: Secretory otitis media and its sequelae (Churchill Livingstone, New York 1979).

187 Sade, J.: Retraction pockets and attic cholesteatomas. Acta oto-rhino-lar. belg. 34: 62–84 (1980).

188 Sade, J.; Avrahma, S.; Brown, M.: The dynamics of atelectic ears and retraction pockets; in Cholesteatoma and mastoid surgery (Kugler, Amsterdam 1982).

189 Sade, J.; Berco, E.: Bone destruction in chronic otitis media: a histopathological study. J. Lar. Otol. 88: 413–422 (1974).

190 Sade, J.; Halevy, A.: The aetiology of bone destruction in chronic otitis media. J. Lar. Otol. 88: 139–143 (1974).

191 Sade, J.; Halevy, A.: The natural history of chronic otitis media. J. Lar. Otol. 90: 743–751 (1976).

192 Sakai, M.; Mikaye, H.; Shinkawa, A.; Mahapatra, A.K.; Chienc, M.: Assessment of postoperative hearing in 528 middle ear and mastoid surgeries (Tokai University Hospital, Tokai).

193 Sakai, M.; Miyake, H.; Shinkawa, A.: Tissue culture studies on migratory property of cholesteatoma matrix and external canal skin; in Cholesteatoma and mastoid surgery (Kugler, Amsterdam 1982).

194 Sanna, M.: Management of labyrinthine fistulae; in Surgery and pathology of the middle ear (Nijhoff, Antwerp 1985).

195 Sanna, M.; Jemmi, G.; Bacciu, S.: La scelta della tecnica nel trattamento chirurgico del colesteatoma nell'infanzia. Annali Lar. Otol. Rinol. Faring. 75: 157 (1976).

196 Sauvage, J.P.: Etude anatomo-chirurgicale de la région du sinus tympani. Conséquences pratiques dans le traitement chirurgical de l'otite chronique et de ses séquelles; thèse Paris (1974).

197 Schuknecht, H.F.: Pathology of the ear (Harvard University Press, Cambridge 1974).

198 Schwartz, R.H.; Linde, R.E.: Iatrogenic implantation cholesteatoma: an unusual complication of tympanostomy tubes. J. Pediat. 94: 432–433 (1979).

199 Schwartz, M.: Das Cholesteatom im Gehörgang und im Mittelohr: Pathogenese, Diagnose, Therapie (Thieme, Stuttgart 1966).
200 Severeid, L.R.: Development of cholesteatoma in children with cleft palate. 1st Int. Conf. on Middle Ear Cholesteatoma, Iowa 1977 (Aesculapius, Birmingham 1977).
201 Sheehy, J.L.: Management of cholesteatoma in children. Adv. Oto-Rhino-Laryng., vol. 23, p. 58 (Karger, Basel 1958).
202 Sheehy, J.L.: Intact canal wall tympanoplasty with mastoidectomy. Laryngoscope 77: 1502 (1967).
203 Sheehy, J.L.: The intact canal wall technique in management of aural cholesteatoma. J. Lar. Otol. 84: 1–31 (1970).
204 Sheehy, J.L.: Plastic sheeting in tympanoplasty. Laryngoscope 83: 1144 (1973).
205 Sheehy, J.L.: Recurrent and residual disease in cholesteatoma surgery. Clin. Otolaryngol. 3: 393–403 (1978).
206 Sheehy, J.L.: Management of the labyrinthine fistula. Clin. Otolaryngol. 3: 405–414 (1978).
207 Sheehy, J.L.: Cholesteatoma surgery in children. Acta oto-rhino-lar. belg. 34: 98–106 (1980).
208 Sheehy, J.L.: Surgical treatment of cholesteatoma at the otologic medical group: residual and recurrent operations (on 307 revisions); in Cholesteatoma and mastoid surgery (Kugler, Amsterdam 1982).
209 Sheehy, J.L.: Tympanoplasty with mastoidectomy: present status. Clin. Otolaryngol. 8: 391–403 (1983).
210 Sheehy, J.L.; Brackmann, D.E.; Graham, M.D.: Cholesteatoma surgery: recurrent and residual disease. Ann. Otol. 86: 451 (1971).
211 Sheehy, J.L.; Brackmann, D.E.; Graham, M.D.: Complications of cholesteatoma – a report of 1,024 cases. 1st Int. Conf. on Middle Ear Cholesteatoma, Iowa 1977 (Aesculapius, Birmingham 1977).
212 Sheehy, J.L.; Brackmann, D.E.; Graham, M.D.: Cholesteatoma surgery: residual and recurrent disease. A review of 1,024 cases. Ann. Otol. 86: 451–462 (1977).
213 Sheehy, J.L.; Crabtree, J.A.: Tympanoplasty – staging the operation. Laryngoscope 83: 1594 (1973).
214 Sheehy, J.L.; Robinson, J.V.: Revision tympanoplasty: residual and recurrent cholesteatoma. A report on 272 intact canal wall revisions; in Cholesteatoma and mastoid surgery (Kugler, Amsterdam 1982).
215 Sheehy, J.L.; Robinson, J.V.: Cholesteatoma surgery at the otologic medical group. Am. J. Otol. 3: 209–215 (1982).
216 Smith, R.; Moran, W.B.: Tympanic membrane keratome (cholesteatoma) in children with no prior otologic surgery. Laryngoscope 87: 237–245 (1977).
217 Smyth, G.D.L.: Postoperative cholesteatoma in combined-approach tympanoplasty – 15-year report on tympanoplasty. Part 1. J. Lar. Otol. 90: 597–622 (1976).
218 Smyth, G.D.L.: Postoperative cholesteatoma. 1st Int. Conf. on Middle Ear Cholesteatoma, Iowa 1977 (Aesculapius, Birmingham 1977).
219 Smyth, G.D.L.: Chronic ear disease. Monographs in clinical otolaryngology (Churchill Livingstone, Edinburgh 1980).
220 Smyth, G.D.L.: Tympanoplasty in children. Am. J. Otol. 1: 199–205 (1980).
221 Smyth, G.D.L.: Practical suggestions on the surgical management of the cholesteatomatous ear. Laryngoscope 92: 456–457 (1982).

222 Smyth, G.D.L.: Cholesteatoma surgery: the influence of the canal wall. Laryngo-
     scope *95:* 92–96 (1985).
223 Smyth, G.D.L.; England, R.M.; Gibson, R.; Kerr, A.G.: Posterior tympanotomy:
     its importance in combined-approach tympanoplasty. J. Lar. Otol. *81:* 69 (1967).
224 Smyth, G.D.L.; Hassard, T.H.: The evolution of policies in the surgical treatment
     of acquired cholesteatoma of the tubotympanic cleft. J. Lar. Otol. *95:* 767–773
     (1981).
225 Sobol, S.M. et al.: Intramembranous and mesotympanic cholesteatomas associated
     with an intact tympanic membrane in children. Ann. Otol. *4:* 312–317 (1980).
226 Sourdille, M.: Trépanation mastoïdienne élargie, atticotomie transmastoïdienne;
     thèse Paris (1915).
227 Steinbach, E.: The innert tympanic cell proliferation theory; in Cholesteatoma and
     mastoid surgery (Kugler, Amsterdam 1982).
228 Sterkers, J.M.: Cholestéatectomie reconstructive. Conservation du conduit. Ferme-
     ture immédiate. Résultats préliminaires dans 25 cas. Annls. Oto-lar. *84:* 263–270
     (1967).
229 Sterkers, J.M.: Facial nerve injuries in the middle ear surgery; in Surgery and pa-
     thology of the middle ear (Nijhoff, Antwerp 1985).
230 Sterkers, J.M.; Sterkers, O.: Cholestéatectomies reconstructives. Technique et ré-
     sultats 12 ans après. Annls. Oto-lar. *97:* 29–34 (1980).
231 Sterkers, J.M.; Sterkers, O.: Cholestéatome et os, extensions pétreuses. Acta oto-
     rhino-lar. belg. *34:* 85–97 (1980).
232 Sterkers, J.M.; Sterkers, O.: Cholestéatomes congénitaux du rocher. Annls. Oto-
     lar. *97:* 579–589 (1980).
233 Strauss, P.: Le traitement chirurgical du cholestéatome: choix entre technique ou-
     verte ou fermée. J. fr. ORL *32:* 578–579 (1982).
234 Thomas, A.: De la tympanotomie postérieure à la cavité autonettoyante; thèse
     Nancy (1975).
235 Thomsen, J.; Bretlau, P.; Jorgensen, M.B.; Kristensen, J.K.: Bone resorption in
     chronic otitis media. 1st Int. Conf. on Middle Ear Cholesteatoma, Iowa 1977 (Aes-
     culapius, Birmingham 1977).
236 Tomoda, K.; Morli, S.; Yamashta, T.; Kumazawa, T.: Histologic architecture of
     submucosal connective tissues in human Eustachian tube. Archs Otolar. *232:* 57–63
     (1981).
237 Tos, M.: Results of tympanoplasty with modified radical mastoidectomy. Acta oto-
     lar. *74:* 61 (1972).
238 Tos, M.: Treatment of labyrnthine fistulae by closed technique. ORL *37:* 41–47
     (1975).
239 Tos, M.: Operative therapy for chronic otitis media and middle ear cholesteatoma
     with preservation of the posterior auditory canal wall (intact canal wall technique).
     HNO *26:* 217–223 (1978).
240 Tos, M.: Pathology of the ossicular chain in various chronic middle ear disease. J.
     Lar. Otol. *93:* 769–780 (1979).
241 Tos, M.: Treatment of cholesteatoma in children. A long-term study of results. Am.
     J. Otol. *4:* 189–197 (1983).
242 Tos, M.: Modification of combined-approach tympanoplasty in attic cholestea-
     toma. Archs Otolar. *108:* 772–778 (1982).

243 Tos, M.: Short- and long-term results with musculoplasty in cholesteatomatous ears; in Cholesteatoma and mastoid surgery (Kugler, Amsterdam 1982).

244 Tumarkin, A.: On the nature and significance of hypocellularity of the mastoid. J. Lar. Otol *73:* 34–44 (1959).

245 Van de Heyning, P.H.; Marquet, J.F.E.: Eradication of cholesteatoma; in Surgery and pathology of the middle ear (Nijhoff, Antwerp 1985).

246 Vaneecloo, F.M.; Christiaens, J.L.; Dhaens, J.; Burny, A.; Piquet, J.J.; Laine, E.: Abcès du cerveau otogènes. Aspects actuels du traitement chirurgical otologique. Revue Oto-Neuro-Ophtal. *53:* 363–370 (1981).

247 Verhoeven, L.: Le traitement du cholestéatome par aspiration trans-méatique. Revue Lar. Otol. Rhinol. *3:* 232 (1961).

248 Waggershauser, C.P.: Mastoid pneumatization and middle ear disease; in Junker, Arnold, Physiology and pathophysiology of Eustachian tube and middle ear (Thieme, Stuttgart 1980).

249 Walsh, T.E.; Cavelmi, W.P.; Ogura, J.H.: The effect of cholesteatosis on bone. Ann. Otol. *60:* 1100–1113 (1951).

250 Wayoff, M.; Bremond, G.; Berezin, A.: Otites moyennes chroniques. EMC ORL, Paris 20.095 Al0, A20 (1975).

251 Wayoff, M.; Bremond, G.; Friot, J.M.; Magnan, J.P.: Les fistules du canal semi-circulaire externe. J.fr. ORL *26:* 49–60 (1977).

252 Wayoff, M.; Chobaut, J.C.; Simon, C.; Jacquot, M.: Oreille moyenne et division palatine (à propos de 230 observations). J. fr. ORL *29:* 10 (1980).

253 Wayoff, M.; Friot, J.M.: Analysis of 100 cases of fistulas of the external semicircular canal. 1st Int. Conf. on Middle Ear Cholesteatoma, Iowa 1977 (Aesculapius, Birmingham 1977).

254 Wayoff, M.; Thomas, A.; Chobaut, J.C.; Simon, C.: La cavité mastoïdienne auto-nettoyante. J. fr. ORL *28:* 5 (1979).

255 Weinberg, J.; Sade, J.: Post-operative cholesteatoma occurrence through the posterior wall. J. Lar. Otol. *85:* 1189 (1971).

256 Weinberg, J.; Sade, J.: Posterior wall atrophy: a late silent complication of the CAT operation; in Cholesteatoma and mastoid surgery (Kugler, Amsterdam 1982).

257 Wullstein, H.: Operationen zur Verbesserung des Gehöres (Thieme, Stuttgart 1968).

258 Wullstein, H.; Wullstein, S.R.: Cholesteatoma – etiology, nosology and tympanoplasty ORL *42:* 313–335 (1980).

259 Wullstein, S.R.: Die osteoplastische Epitympanotomie und die Pathologie des Mittelohres. Z. Lar. Rhinol. Otol. *52:* 34 (1973).

260 Zechner, G.: Stratified squamous epithelium in retraction pockets and attic cholesteatoma; in Cholesteatoma and mastoid surgery (Kugler, Amsterdam 1982).

261 Zini, C.; Sanna, M.: La tympanotomia posteriore nel trattamento chirurgico delle otomastoiditi croniche. Estratto dagli atti del XX Conventus Societas Latina, Roma 1974.

262 Zini, C.; Sheehy, J.L.; Sanna, M.: Microsurgery of cholesteatoma of the middle ear (Kugler, Amsterdam 1983).

Subject Index